MEDICAL MASTERCLASS

Endocrinology

Disclaimer

Although every effort has been made to ensure that drug doses and other information are presented accurately in this publication, the ultimate responsibility rests with the prescribing physician. Neither the publishers nor the authors can be held responsible for any consequences arising from the use of information contained herein. Any product mentioned in this publication should be used in accordance with the prescribing information prepared by the manufacturers.

The information presented in this publication reflects the opinions of its contributors and should not be taken to represent the policy and views of the Royal College of Physicians of London, unless this is specifically stated.

Every effort has been made by the contributors to contact holders of copyright to obtain permission to reproduce copyright material. However, if any have been inadvertently overlooked, the publisher will be pleased to make the necessary arrangements at the first opportunity.

Medical Masterclass

EDITOR-IN-CHIEF

John D. Firth DM FRCP

Consultant Physician and Nephrologist
Addenbrooke's Hospital
Cambridge

Endocrinology

EDITOR

M. Gurnell BSc Hons MBBS MRCP PhD

Wellcome Training Fellow and Specialist Registrar
Addenbrooke's Hospital
Cambridge

Blackwell
Science

© 2001 Royal College of Physicians of London, 11 St Andrews Place, London NW1 4LE, Registered Charity No. 210508

Published by:
Blackwell Science Ltd
Editorial Offices:
Osney Mead, Oxford OX2 0EL
25 John Street, London WC1N 2BS
23 Ainslie Place, Edinburgh EH3 6AJ
350 Main Street, Malden
   MA 02148-5018, USA
54 University Street, Carlton
   Victoria 3053, Australia
10, rue Casimir Delavigne
   75006 Paris, France

Other Editorial Offices:
Blackwell Wissenschafts-Verlag GmbH
Kurfürstendamm 57
10707 Berlin, Germany

Blackwell Science KK
MG Kodenmacho Building
7–10 Kodenmacho Nihombashi
Chuo-ku, Tokyo 104, Japan

Iowa State University Press
A Blackwell Science Company
2121 S. State Avenue
Ames, Iowa 50014-8300, USA

First published 2001

Set by Graphicraft Limited, Hong Kong
Printed and bound in Italy by
Rotolito Lombarda SpA, Milan

Catalogue records for this title are available from the British Library and the Library of Congress

ISBN 0-632-05869-2 (this book)
   0-632-05567-7 (set)

Commissioning Editors: Mike Stein and Rachel Robson
Project Manager (RCP): Filipa Maia
Editorial Assistant (RCP): Katherine Bowker
Production: Charlie Hamlyn and Jonathan Rowley
Layout and Cover Design: Chris Stone

DISTRIBUTORS

Marston Book Services Ltd
PO Box 269
Abingdon, Oxon OX14 4YN
(*Orders*: Tel: 01235 465500
      Fax: 01235 465555)

USA
Blackwell Science, Inc.
Commerce Place
350 Main Street
Malden, MA 02148-5018
(*Orders*: Tel: 800 759 6102
      781 388 8250
      Fax: 781 388 8255)

Canada
Login Brothers Book Company
324 Saulteaux Crescent
Winnipeg, Manitoba R3J 3T2
(*Orders*: Tel: 204 837 2987)

Australia
Blackwell Science Pty Ltd
54 University Street
Carlton, Victoria 3053
(*Orders*: Tel: 3 9347 0300
      Fax: 3 9347 5001)

For further information on Blackwell Science, visit our website:
www.blackwell-science.com

Contents

List of contributors

Anna Crown MA MB BChir MRCP PhD
Specialist Registrar
Bristol Royal Infirmary
Bristol

Paul D Flynn MA MB BChir MRCP MRCPI PhD
Clinical Lecturer
University of Cambridge
Addenbrooke's Hospital
Cambridge

Mark Gurnell BSc Hons MBBS MRCP PhD
Wellcome Training Fellow and Specialist Registrar
Addenbrooke's Hospital
Cambridge

Mohammed Z Qureshi MBBS MRCP
Staff Physician
Blackpool Victoria Hospital
Blackpool

Foreword

Medical Masterclass is the most innovative and important educational development from the Royal College of Physicians in the last 100 years. Throughout our 480-year history we have pioneered and supported high-quality medicine, and while *Medical Masterclass* continues that tradition, it also represents a quantum leap for the College as it moves into the 21st century.

The effort that the College has put in to improve the Membership Examination, which started 150 years ago and is now run by all three UK Royal Colleges of Physicians, will now be matched by its attention to basic learning in general medicine—the grounding and preparation for the exam.

Teaching and learning for the exam have changed little over the past 50 years, relying on local courses, word-based teaching and commercial courses. *Medical Masterclass* is a completely new approach for those wishing to practise high-quality medicine. It is an imaginative multimedia programme with paper and CD modules covering the major areas of medicine, supported by a website which will provide summaries and links to the latest articles and guidelines, and self-assessment questionnaires with feedback. Its focus is on self-learning, self-assessment and dealing with realistic clinical problems—not just force-feeding facts. The series of interactive case studies on which the modules are based entail making diagnostic and treatment decisions, closely mimicking the situations found in the admission suite or outpatient clinic.

Medical Masterclass has been produced by the RCP's Education Department together with Blackwell Science. It represents a formidable amount of work by Dr John Firth and his team of authors and editors and is set to be the jewel in our crown. It also signals very clearly our intention to lead in the field of learning and to be supportive to our future members. I anticipate the package will also be invaluable for continued learning by our specialist registrars and consultants as part of continuing professional development.

I congratulate our colleagues for this superb product and commend it to you without reservation.

Professor Sir George Alberti
President of the Royal College of Physicians, London

Preface

Medical Masterclass comprises twelve paper-based modules, two CD-ROMs and a companion website. Its aim is to help doctors in their first few years of training to improve their medical skills and knowledge.

The twelve paper-based modules are divided as follows: two cover the scientific background to medicine, one is devoted to general clinical issues, one to emergency medicine and practical procedures, and eight cover the range of medical specialities. Medicine is often fairly straightforward when the diagnosis is clear, but patients rarely come to their doctor and say 'I've got Hodgkin's disease': they have lumps. The core material of each of the clinical specialities is defined by case presentations in the first part of each module: how do you approach the man who has lumps? Structured concise notes on specific diseases follow later. All practising doctors know that medicine is much more than knowing lots of facts about diseases: how do you tell someone they've got cancer? How do you decide when to stop treatment? Most medical texts say little about these issues: *Medical Masterclass* does not avoid them, nor does it talk in vague and abstract terms.

The two CD-ROMs each contain 30 interactive cases requiring diagnosis and treatment. The format is remarkably close to real life: you see the patient and are told the story; you have to decide how to investigate and treat; but you can't see all the results before you start to make decisions!

The companion website, which will be regularly updated, includes literature and guideline updates and review, and self-assessment questions. How much do you know, and are you improving? You will see how your score compares with your previous attempts, and also how your performance compares with others who have logged on to the site.

The *Medical Masterclass* is produced by the Education Department of the Royal College of Physicians of London and published by Blackwell Science. It is not a crammer for the MRCP exam and is not written by those who set the exam. However, I have no doubt that someone putting effort into learning through the *Medical Masterclass* would be in a strong position to impress the examiners, although I am afraid that success—like much else in medicine and in life—cannot be guaranteed.

John Firth
Editor-in-Chief

Acknowledgements

Medical Masterclass has been produced by a team. The names of those who have written and edited material are clearly indicated elsewhere, but without the efforts of many other people *Medical Masterclass* would not exist at all. These include Professor Lesley Rees and Mrs Winnie Wade from the Education Department of the Royal College of Physicians of London, who initiated the project; Dr Mike Stein and Dr Andy Robinson from Medschool.com and Blackwell Science respectively, who have enthusiastically supported it from the beginning; and Ms Filipa Maia and Ms Katherine Bowker, who have run the office with splendid efficiency and induced authors and editors to perform to a schedule rarely achieved. I and the whole of the team of editors and authors are immensely grateful to all of these people for the energy that they have poured into *Medical Masterclass* in various ways.

John Firth
Editor-in-Chief

The authors and editor would also like to thank the following people for their help in the preparation of this module: Dr N. Antoun, Addenbrooke's Hospital, Cambridge, Professor K. Chatterjee, Addenbrooke's Hospital, Cambridge, Dr J. Compston, University of Cambridge Department of Medicine, Addenbrooke's Hospital, Cambridge, Dr E.C. Crowne, Bristol Childrens Hospital, Dr E. Gurnell, Addenbrooke's Hospital, Cambridge and Dr J. Kabala, Bristol Royal Infirmary.

Mark Gurnell, Paul Flynn, Anna Crown,
Mohammed Qureshi

Key features

We have created a range of icon boxes to help you identify key information and to make learning easier and more enjoyable. Here is a brief explanation:

Clinical pointer

This icon highlights important information to be noted.

Further information

This icon indicates the source of further information and reference.

Hints

This icon highlights useful hints, tips and mnemonics.

Key points

This icon is used to highlight points of particular importance.

Quote

This icon indicates useful or interesting citations from notable individuals, including well-known physicians.

Think about

This icon indicates what the reader should reflect on after having read a passage from the text.

Warning/Hazard

This icon is used to indicate common or important drug interactions, pitfalls of practical procedures, or when to take symptoms or signs particularly seriously.

Endocrinology

AUTHORS:
A. Crown, P. Flynn, M. Gurnell, M. Qureshi

EDITOR:
M. Gurnell

EDITOR-IN-CHIEF:
J.D. Firth

Clinical presentations

1.1 Hyponatraemia

Case history

A 72-year-old woman, previously well apart from mild hypertension, has been admitted comatose to Accident and Emergency (A&E). A computed tomography (CT) scan of her head has shown no abnormality, but her serum sodium is 112 mmol/L.

Clinical approach

 The unconscious patient

In a comatose patient, always check a blood glucose level at the bedside before proceeding any further, even if there appears to be another explanation for the coma. Untreated hypoglycaemia can result in serious neurological sequelae and is easily corrected with 25 or 50% dextrose.

The first priority is clearly to ensure safe management of the unconscious patient, the next is to consider the broad differential diagnosis of hyponatraemia. It is likely that the two problems are connected, but this is not certain. Is the patient hypovolaemic, euvolaemic or hypervolaemic? Are there clues to any of the diagnoses listed in Tables 1 and 2 and Fig. 1?

History of the presenting problem

This woman is unconscious, hence any history will need to be obtained from a relative or partner who has accompanied the patient, and as much as possible will need to be gleaned from the GP's letter, or through a telephone call to the GP (if available). Given the wide differential of both coma and hyponatraemia, directed questions should be guided by your initial clinical observations.

General

The approach to the patient who is comatose is described in *Emergency medicine*, Section 1.26, but it is essential to get the following information:
- Who found her?
- What were the circumstances?
- When was she last seen before that, and did she appear to be well?
- Is there any possibility that she has taken an overdose?

Table 1 Causes of hyponatraemia.

Volume status	Total body water	Total extracellular sodium	Primary problem	Example
Hypovolaemic	Low	Even lower	Renal	Diuretics Sodium-losing renal disease Mineralocorticoid deficiency
			Non-renal	Vomiting Diarrhoea Burns Excessive sweating
Euvolaemic	Normal/slight excess	Reduced/normal	—	SIADH Glucocorticoid deficiency Hypothyroidism 'Sick cells'
Hypervolaemic	Great excess	Excess	Renal Non-renal	Acute/chronic renal failure Cardiac failure Cirrhosis/liver failure Nephrotic syndrome

SIADH, syndrome of inappropriate antidiuretic hormone.

Source of ADH	Type of problem	Example
Ectopic ADH production	Malignancy	Small cell lung cancer
Inappropriate pituitary ADH secretion	Malignancy	Lung cancer, lymphoma
	Inflammatory lung disease	Pneumonia, lung abscess
	Neurological disease	Meningitis, head injury, subdural haematoma, postsurgery
	Drugs	Antidepressants (tricyclics, SSRIs), carbamazepine, chlorpropamide, phenothiazines, (e.g. chlorpromazine), vincristine, cyclophosphamide, ecstasy*
	Postoperative*	—
	Others	Hypothyroidism, anterior pituitary insufficiency, porphyria

Table 2 Causes of the syndrome of inappropriate antidiuretic hormone (SIADH).

*Other factors, i.e. drinking of water or iatrogenic 5% dextrose administration, contribute to the development of hyponatraemia.
ADH, antidiuretic hormone; SSRIs, selective serotonin reuptake inhibitors.

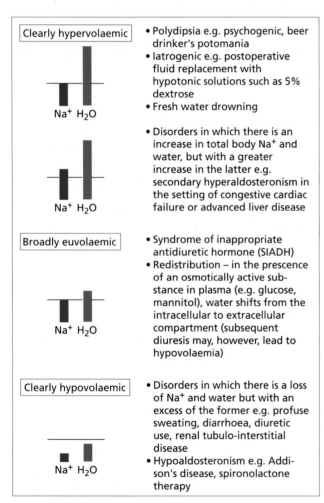

- Clearly hypervolaemic
  Na^+ H_2O
  - Polydipsia e.g. psychogenic, beer drinker's potomania
  - Iatrogenic e.g. postoperative fluid replacement with hypotonic solutions such as 5% dextrose
  - Fresh water drowning

  Na^+ H_2O
  - Disorders in which there is an increase in total body Na^+ and water, but with a greater increase in the latter e.g. secondary hyperaldosteronism in the setting of congestive cardiac failure or advanced liver disease

- Broadly euvolaemic
  Na^+ H_2O
  - Syndrome of inappropriate antidiuretic hormone (SIADH)
  - Redistribution – in the prescence of an osmotically active substance in plasma (e.g. glucose, mannitol), water shifts from the intracellular to extracellular compartment (subsequent diuresis may, however, lead to hypovolaemia)

- Clearly hypovolaemic
  Na^+ H_2O
  - Disorders in which there is a loss of Na^+ and water but with an excess of the former e.g. profuse sweating, diarrhoea, diuretic use, renal tubulo-interstitial disease
  - Hypoaldosteronism e.g. Addison's disease, spironolactone therapy

Fig. 1 Hyponatraemia and volume status.

- If anyone who knows anything about the woman is available, then ask for details that might give a clue as to why she is hyponatraemic and why she might be comatose (if the two are different).

Neurological

The neurological history is clearly of prime importance in someone who is comatose, since a neurological problem could cause coma in its own right, or in this case via hyponatraemia induced by syndrome of inappropriate antidiuretic hormone (SIADH) secretion. Ask about:
- head injury
- fluctuating consciousness—suggestive of subdural haematoma
- headaches—especially with features of raised intracranial pressure
- symptoms suggestive of meningeal irritation—neck stiffness, photophobia.

Reasons for hyponatraemia

Think of the conditions listed in Tables 1 and 2 as you take the history. Enquire about the following.

Features of malignancy

Has there been weight loss, unexplained fever, night sweats, pruritus? Could this woman have lung cancer complicated by SIADH? What are her current or past smoking habits? Have there been features of lung cancer (e.g. cough, haemoptysis, dyspnoea, pleuritic chest pain), or symptoms of pulmonary inflammation (e.g. purulent cough, dyspnoea)?

Fluid loss and fluid intake

Has the woman had diarrhoea or vomiting? What has she been drinking, and how much? Psychogenic polydipsia is extremely unlikely in a woman of this age, most commonly being seen in young psychiatric patients when excessive intake is frequently concealed.

Drug history

Diuretics are a very common cause of hyponatraemia and this woman has hypertension. Is she taking a diuretic? Enquire also about drugs associated with SIADH (Table 2), angiotensin converting enzyme (ACE) inhibitors, exogenous steroids and nephrotoxins. If no other explanation for hyponatraemia emerges, it might even be appropriate to ask someone to go round to her house and bring back all her bottles of pills.

Other aspects

Is there a history of cardiac, renal or liver failure, or of nephrotic syndrome? Is it possible that there is an endocrine cause of hyponatraemia? Ask about the following:
• hypothyroidism—ask about weight gain, cold intolerance, constipation (see Section 2.3, p. 67)
• hypopituitarism—enquire specifically about symptoms of hypogonadism, hypothyroidism and hypoadrenalism (see Section 2.1.7, p. 57)
• Addison's disease—unexplained hyponatraemia in a comatose patient should prompt immediate consideration of hypoadrenalism (see Section 2.2, p. 59)
• porphyria—abdominal pain, neuropathy and preceding psychiatric illness in a younger patient are important clues to the diagnosis (see Section 2.5.2, p. 87).

Examination

In any comatose patient the immediate priorities are:
• check airway, breathing, circulation: insert oropharyngeal airway if tolerated
• check Glasgow Coma Scale score.

See *Emergency medicine*, Section 1.26, for further information. In this case, pursue the cause of hyponatraemia as follows.

Fluid status

Assessment of volume status

Accurate assessment of volume status is vital in diagnosis of the cause of hyponatraemia. Check carefully for:
• hypovolaemia—the most reliable signs are a low jugular venous pressure and postural hypotension
• hypervolaemia—look for a raised jugular venous pressure, gallop rhythm, pulmonary oedema, peripheral oedema.

General

Look specifically for:
• pyrexia—infection/inflammation

• clubbing—malignancy or pyogenic lung disease
• lymphadenopathy—malignancy
• Horner's syndrome—Pancoast's tumour
• buccal/palmar/generalized pigmentation—Addison's disease
• myxoedematous features—hypothyroidism
• diminished body hair—hypopituitarism.

Other

A full physical examination is required:
• cardiac—is there evidence of heart failure?
• respiratory—look for signs of collapse/consolidation and bronchiectasis
• abdominal—check for features of chronic liver disease or hepatomegaly
• neurological—look for neck stiffness, photophobia, papilloedema or any focal neurological deficits.

Approach to investigation and management

In any comatose patient the immediate priorities are:
• ensure protection of the airway
• give high-flow oxygen by face mask
• exclude hypoglycaemia and opiate toxicity.

See *Emergency Medicine*, Section 1.26, for further information. This woman has already had a CT scan, which is normal, and attention is clearly focused on her hyponatraemia.

Investigations

Beware factitious hyponatraemia

Although highly unlikely in this case, factitious hyponatraemia (e.g. sampling from a 'drip' arm) and pseudohyponatraemia (e.g. in the context of gross hyperlipidaemia) should be excluded before embarking on more detailed investigations, particularly if the serum sodium is extremely low and yet the patient seems well!

Routine blood tests

Check full blood count (anaemia, leukocytosis, low haematocrit), urea and electrolytes (dehydration, hypoadrenalism), glucose, liver biochemistry (intrinsic liver disease, malignancy), calcium (malignancy), phosphate (renal tubular defects), free thyroxine (FT_4) and thyroid-stimulating hormone (TSH) (primary or secondary hypothyroidism).

PAIRED PLASMA (OR SERUM) AND URINE OSMOLALITIES

A key investigation in the diagnosis of SIADH, which must be supplemented by measurement of a 'spot' urinary sodium concentration, since SIADH cannot be diagnosed in the face of a low urinary sodium concentration. The latter indicates that the kidney is conserving sodium because of 'real' or 'perceived' intravascular volume depletion, which will stimulate antidiuretic hormone (ADH) release and water retention that is appropriate for the defence of intravascular volume, although inappropriate for regulation of osmolality, i.e. with reference to Table 1:

• urinary sodium concentration is low (<10 mmol/L) in non-renal causes of both hypovolaemic and hypervolaemic hyponatraemia

• urinary sodium concentration is high (>20 mmol/L) in renal causes of hypovolaemic and hypervolaemic hyponatraemia, and in normovolaemic hyponatraemia

• intermediate urinary sodium concentrations (10–20 mmol/L) are difficult to interpret but should probably be regarded as indicating non-renal causes of hyponatraemia.

Criteria for the diagnosis of SIADH

• Clinically euvolaemic
• Decreased plasma sodium and osmolality
• Inappropriately high urinary sodium concentration and osmolality
• Normal adrenal, renal and thyroid function

Calculation of plasma osmolality

The measured plasma osmolality can be compared with a calculated value to exclude the presence of other osmotically active substance(s) in plasma:

Calculated osmolality = $\{([Na^+] + [K^+]) \times 2\} + [urea] + [glucose]$

This is most often useful in the context of poisoning, e.g. ethylene glycol (antifreeze) overdose (see *Emergency medicine*, Section 1.19).

Other investigations

These will be determined by your clinical findings:
• CT head scan is normal in this case
• chest radiograph and lumbar puncture may be appropriate.

Management

Treatment of acute adrenal insufficiency in an emergency

If there is any suggestion of acute adrenal insufficiency, treatment with hydrocortisone (100 mg i.v.) must not be delayed. A serum sample should be saved for subsequent cortisol estimation (see Section 2.2, p. 59).

Specific management will depend on the underlying condition, and this should be treated vigorously whenever possible.

Chronic asymptomatic hyponatraemia

Unless there is definite evidence to the contrary it should be assumed that hyponatraemia is chronic (i.e. >48 h duration) and that cerebral adaptation has occurred. If there are no symptoms, plasma sodium should always be corrected over days, and there is no indication whatever for attempts to raise the serum sodium rapidly.

• If hypovolaemic with no major symptoms from hyponatraemia—give i.v. 0.9% saline replacement cautiously until volume is restored, then restrict water intake

• If euvolaemic or hypervolaemic with no major symptoms from hyponatraemia—restrict water to 1000 mL per day or less, giving this as ice in aliquots through the day and ensuring that swabs are available to moisten the mouth. In those cases where the underlying cause cannot be corrected (e.g. lung cancer) demeclocycline may be useful, inducing a partial nephrogenic DI and reversing the inappropriate antidiuresis.

Acute symptomatic hyponatraemia

If there are neurological complications attributable to hyponatraemia, as are present in this case, then urgent treatment is required, but even here it is important not to undertake too rapid a correction, which can cause irreversible and often fatal central pontine myelinolysis. Outside hospital it is rare for hyponatraemia to develop suddenly, but within hospital this can happen, almost invariably due to inappropriate i.v. administration of large volumes of 5% dextrose to patients who are unable to excrete water normally, e.g. in the immediate post-operative period. Treatment is as follows:

• 'normal' (0.9%) saline is hypertonic relative to the patient's plasma: twice normal (1.8%) saline should be reserved for those cases where there is a need to avoid excess volume expansion

• aim to correct the plasma sodium by no more than 0.5–1.0 mmol/L per hour (and by a maximum of 25 mmol/L in 48 h), with frequent estimation of plasma sodium and adjustment of infusion rate as required (Table 3)

• infusion of hypertonic solutions must be stopped once the plasma sodium is between 125 and 130 mmol/L, and should be stopped sooner if neurological symptoms have improved: they must not be continued until sodium concentration is 'back to normal'.

Correction of hyponatraemia with hypertonic saline

Assuming:
- target plasma [Na⁺] = 130 mmol/L
- correction rate of 1 mmol/L per hour
- 150 mmol/L sodium in normal saline and 300 mmol/L in twice normal saline.

Then:

Table 3 Calculating infusion rate.

1	Measure plasma [Na⁺]	y (mmol/L)
2	Estimate total body water, i.e. 35–60% body weight (kg)	x (L) (35% in elderly obese women, 60% in young lean men)
3	Subtract the patient's plasma sodium from 130. This indicates both: • Required correction of plasma sodium in mmol/L, and • Minimum number of hours over which correction should occur	$130 - y$
4	Calculate total body sodium deficit	$(130 - y) \cdot x$ (mmol)
5	Calculate volume of saline required: Normal saline Twice normal saline	$(130 - y) \cdot x / 150$ (L) $(130 - y) \cdot x / 300$ (L)
6	Multiply by 1000 to give the number of mL saline required	
7	Calculate infusion rate (mL/h)	Volume required (mL)/$130 - y$ (h)

Giving hypertonic saline in hyponatraemia

- Infusion of hypertonic saline is dangerous and should be restricted to those cases where hyponatraemia is causing neurological sequelae such as altered conscious level or fits. In these circumstances the plasma sodium will be <120 mmol/L: if not consider other causes of coma
- Hypertonic saline should not be given where there is an increase in total body sodium with oedema, e.g. in advanced liver disease.

See *Emergency medicine*, Section 1.18.
Gill G, Leese G. Hyponatraemia: biochemical and clinical perspectives. *Postgrad Med J* 1998; 74: 516–523.

1.2 Hypercalcaemia

Case history

A 54-year-old postmenopausal woman presents with a history of a renal calculus. Initial investigations have shown a serum calcium of 2.8 mmol/L.

Table 4 Composition of urinary stones and their frequency.

Stone type	Frequency (%)
Calcium oxalate/phosphate	40
Calcium oxalate	25
Triple phosphate (struvite)	15
Calcium phosphate	5–10
Uric acid	5–10
Cystine	3

Clinical approach

Most urinary tract calculi contain calcium (Table 4), and the majority of patients (~65%) have idiopathic hypercalciuria, but some 5% have underlying hypercalcaemia, as in this case. Ideally, this should be confirmed on an uncuffed venous sample. Although the differential diagnosis of hypercalcaemia is broad (Table 5), the presence of a renal stone usually implies that the hypercalcaemia is long-standing and therefore unlikely to be secondary to malignancy. The most likely diagnosis here is primary hyperparathyroidism.

History of the presenting problem

Symptoms of hypercalcaemia

These usually occur when the serum calcium exceeds 3 mmol/L, and comprise thirst and polyuria, constipation and anorexia, general malaise, depression and anxiety. More severe hypercalcaemia can lead to vomiting, severe dehydration, confusion and even coma (see Section 2.5.7, p. 95 and 2.5.8, p. 97).

Complications of hypercalcaemia

Long-standing hypercalcaemia, usually caused by hyperparathyroidism, can be associated with bone disease in addition to urolithiasis. Is there a history of bone pain or pathological fracture?

Cause of hypercalcaemia

A full drug history should be taken, asking specifically about:
- lithium—which potentiates the effects of parathyroid hormone (PTH)
- thiazide diuretics—which both reduce urinary calcium excretion and potentiate the effects of PTH
- vitamin D intake
- milk, alkali, antacids.

The symptoms of sarcoidosis, tuberculosis, Addison's disease, phaeochromocytoma and thyrotoxicosis should also be sought as these can occasionally cause hypercalcaemia. In patients presenting acutely, careful attention should be

Table 5 Causes of hypercalcaemia.*

Frequency	Type of disorder	Example
Common	Primary hyperparathyroidism	—
	Malignancy	Carcinoma with skeletal metastases, e.g. breast, lung
		Carcinoma without skeletal metastases, i.e. humoral hypercalcaemia of malignancy
		Haematological disorders, e.g. myeloma
Less common	Vitamin D toxicity	Consumption of medicines/compounds containing vitamin D
	Vitamin D 'sensitivity'	Granulomatous disorders, e.g. sarcoidosis
	Excess calcium intake	Milk–alkali syndrome
	Reduced calcium excretion	Thiazide diuretics, lithium
		Familial hypocalciuric hypercalcaemia
	Endocrine/metabolic	Thyrotoxicosis
		Adrenal failure
		Phaeochromocytoma
	Other	Acute renal failure
		Long-term immobility
		Tertiary hyperparathyroidism

*Note that artefactual hypercalcaemia is common and can be due to venous stasis at phlebotomy, hyperalbuminaemia or hypergammaglobulinaemia.

given to obtaining a history that might support the diagnosis of malignancy (particularly lung) or myeloma.

A family history of hypercalcaemia may suggest the presence of multiple endocrine neoplasia (MEN) (see Section 2.7, p. 115).

Examination

There are few signs of hypercalcaemia *per se*. Occasionally band keratopathy (corneal calcification) may be seen, which is best detected on slit lamp examination. Severe hypercalcaemia frequently leads to dehydration. Examination should be directed towards:
- assessing for signs of volume depletion, i.e. postural hypotension, low jugular venous pressure
- establishing the underlying cause, e.g. malignancy (particularly checking the breasts and the lungs), lymphoma (looking carefully for lymphadenopathy or splenomegaly), sarcoidosis, tuberculosis.

Approach to investigation and management

For details of the approach to the investigation and management of renal calculi see *Nephrology*, Sections 1.13 and 2.6.2.

Investigations

Full details of the approach to the investigation of hypercalcaemia are outlined in Section 2.5.8, p. 96. In primary hyperparathyroidism the serum calcium level is almost invariably elevated, whilst phosphate is low; serum PTH is high, or inappropriately normal. In all other causes of hypercalcaemia (except tertiary hyperparathyroidism) PTH is suppressed.

Management

The management of hypercalcaemia (both acute and chronic) is covered in detail in Section 2.5.8, p. 96. Specific treatment will depend on the underlying disorder.

Primary hyperparathyroidism

With a calcium level that is only mildly elevated at 2.8, and in the absence of symptoms of polyuria and polydipsia or confusion, it is debatable whether any immediate specific treatment is required, other than ensuring adequate hydration. In the longer term, however, given that there is a history of urolithiasis, definitive treatment should be offered. In the case of a solitary parathyroid adenoma the preferred option is surgical excision. The only controversy is whether preoperative imaging should be performed, for example with ^{99m}Tc-sestamibi scanning; currently this depends on local practice. Postoperatively transient hypocalcaemia may occur, which can be treated with 10% calcium gluconate i.v. in the acute setting, or with a combination of vitamin D and calcium supplements in milder cases.

 See *Emergency medicine*, Section 1.18; *Haematology*, Sections 1.15 and 2.2.1; *Nephrology*, Sections 1.13, 1.14, 2.6.2 and 2.7.1. Bushinsky DA, Monk RD. Calcium. *N Engl J Med* 1998; 352: 306–311.

1.3 Polyuria

Case history

A 22-year-old man is referred from the orthopaedic wards with polyuria.

Clinical approach

Polyuria is defined as the passage of an abnormally large volume of urine, and should be distinguished from frequency of micturition. It is usually taken to indicate the passage of at least 3 L in 24 h, a useful surrogate marker being nocturia on two to three occasions each night. If polyuria is confirmed, there is a large number of possible causes (Table 6), and the history, clinical examination and initial investigations should be used to direct more detailed study. In essence, diabetes mellitus (DM), chronic renal failure (CRF) and other causes of an osmotic diuresis should be excluded prior to distinguishing between diabetes insipidus (DI) and compulsive water intoxication.

History of the presenting problem

The first requirement is to be sure that polyuria really is present. If there is any doubt at all about this, a 24-h urinary collection should be performed: if all the urine fits in one of the standard containers, then the problem may be frequency, but not polyuria.

Fluid intake

In this case, check the drips and fluid balance charts: how much fluid is being infused and what is the recorded urinary output? Also check the drug charts: has he just been given a diuretic?! In all cases take a careful history of drinking behaviour: exactly what did the patient have to drink yesterday, what on a typical day, and why did they drink it? Begin when they wake up, and work through the day. In an outpatient context, it is not at all uncommon for someone referred with polyuria to have drunk several cups of tea or coffee, two cans of fizzy drink and 0.5 L of water before lunch, the reason being recognized by them as 'habit' rather than thirst, but often also driven by a belief that it is good to 'keep the kidneys flushed'. However, even in cases where it seems immediately apparent that excessive fluid intake out of habit is the reason for polyuria, it is appropriate to look for evidence on history, examination and simple testing of the other conditions listed in Table 6, since it can be difficult to know which came first—the polydipsia or the polyuria; the chicken or the egg?

Osmotic diuresis

Exclude causes of an osmotic diuresis. Ask specifically about:
• DM—is there a personal or family history of DM? Are there symptoms of hyperglycaemia (lassitude, increased appetite, weight loss) and, if appropriate, of diabetic complications (see Section 2.6, p. 100)? A blood glucose test strip may, of course, confirm the diagnosis of hyperglycaemia immediately
• CRF—uncommon in this age group and symptoms are non-specific. The renal function tests will make or refute this diagnosis. If CRF is present, then clearly this will require explanation (see *Nephrology*, Sections 1.5 and 2.1).

Diabetes insipidus

Table 7 lists many of the causes of DI and questions should be directed at screening for these disorders. For example, when considering pituitary dysfunction, a history of head injury (as occurred in this case, following a motorcycle accident), surgery or radiotherapy should be sought, together with evidence of raised intracranial pressure (headaches, especially first thing in the morning) or of anterior pituitary failure (lassitude, weight gain, cold intolerance, constipation, diminished libido).

Table 6 Aetiology of polyuria.

Problem	Example
Osmotic diuresis	DM (glucose) Chronic renal failure (urea) Intravenous infusions (saline, mannitol) Diuretics
Abnormal renal tubular water handling	DI: pituitary, nephrogenic
Excessive fluid intake	Habitual excessive drinking (non-psychiatric) Psychogenic polydipsia, Iatrogenic

DI, diabetes insipidus; DM, diabetes mellitus.

Table 7 Causes of diabetes insipidus.

Pituitary	Idiopathic Familial, e.g. DIDMOAD Post-head injury Cranial or pituitary surgery/radiotherapy Tumour, e.g. craniopharyngioma, metastases (breast, lung) Granulomata, e.g. sarcoidosis, tuberculosis, histiocytosis Infections, e.g. meningitis, encephalitis Vascular, e.g. aneurysm
Nephrogenic	Familial (X-linked) Renal disorders, e.g. tubulointerstitial disease, obstructive uropathy Electrolyte imbalance, e.g. hypercalcaemia, hypokalaemia Drugs, e.g. lithium, demeclocycline

DIDMOAD, diabetes insipidus, diabetes mellitus, optic atrophy, deafness.

Psychogenic polydipsia

Compulsive water intoxication (rather than simply habitual non-psychiatric excessive drinking) is likely to be concealed and details may need to be sought from a relative, partner or carer. It is most commonly seen in those with a history of psychiatric illness.

Examination

Bear in mind the causes of polyuria whilst performing a thorough physical examination. There are likely to be few signs in the newly presenting type 1 diabetic and it would be rare to find diagnostic signs in CRF. Check for:
• evidence of hypopituitarism (see Section 2.1, p. 47)
• signs of local pituitary tumour expansion, including visual field defects (classically bitemporal hemianopia)
• DI, DM, optic atrophy, deafness (DIDMOAD). This is very rare, but you'll never make the diagnosis if you don't consider it!

Approach to investigation and management

Investigation of polyuria
• Confirm that polyuria is present before embarking on tests
• Exclude osmotic diuresis (high glucose/high urea/mannitol)
• Consider DI—pituitary or nephrogenic
• Consider psychogenic polydipsia.

Investigations

Routine blood tests

These should include a full blood count (anaemia), electrolytes, renal function tests, blood glucose, liver and bone biochemistry (specifically calcium, phosphate and alkaline phosphatase), and thyroid function tests ([TFTs] FT_4 and TSH).

Urinalysis

Check specifically for glycosuria, haematuria and proteinuria.

Chest radiograph

Look for evidence of pulmonary sarcoidosis or tuberculosis.

Further investigations

Having excluded an osmotic basis for polyuria, the diagnosis now rests between DI (pituitary or nephrogenic) and psychogenic polydipsia. Plasma osmolality may be helpful—this is usually:

• lower than 290 mOsm/kg in polydipsia, reflecting volume overload
• greater than normal in DI, reflecting volume depletion.
Formal investigation requires a water deprivation test (see Section 3.3.2, p. 124). If pituitary DI is confirmed, the pituitary and hypothalamus should be imaged by magnetic resonance imaging (MRI) and dynamic tests of pituitary function (see Sections 2.1, p. 47 and 3.1, p. 117) should be considered. Patients with nephrogenic DI require more detailed tests of renal tubular function.

Management

The patient who has simply got into the habit of drinking excessively should be reassured after simple screening that there is nothing seriously wrong and that their urinary volume, and any attendant embarrassment caused by the need for frequent micturition, will be eased if they can gradually wean down the amount of fluid that they drink. Disorders such as DM and CRF will require appropriate treatment.

Pituitary diabetes insipidus

Symptomatic relief may be provided with the synthetic vasopressin analogue desmopressin. This can be administered orally, or more conveniently via a nasal spray (see Section 2.1, p. 47). Any associated anterior pituitary failure should also be treated with appropriate hormone replacement.

Nephrogenic diabetes insipidus

Thiazide diuretics (e.g. hydrochlorothiazide) in combination with mild sodium restriction are often effective. Amiloride may be of benefit, especially in lithium-induced DI.

Psychogenic polydipsia

Polyuria can be controlled by limiting fluid intake, but this is easier said than done. Most patients have a known psychiatric disorder: in those that do not, formal psychiatric input should be considered. However, the reason for trying to restrain drinking and polyuria in this condition needs to be considered. Unless of massive degree, it is likely that the only complication of psychogenic polydipsia is the inconvenience of urinary frequency and reassurance to the patient, relatives and carers that there is no 'serious pathology' may be the limit of useful medical contribution.

Baylis PH. Water and sodium homeostasis and their disorders. In: (eds) *Oxford Textbook of Medicine*, 3rd edn, pp. 3116–3122. Oxford: Oxford University Press, 1996.

1.4 Faints, sweats and palpitations

Case history

A 46-year-old woman presents with recurrent episodes of light-headedness associated with sweating and palpitations. She is finding it increasingly difficult to cope at home, particularly with her 16-year-old daughter who has diabetes mellitus (DM).

Clinical approach

Although the symptoms described may have no clear physical basis and simply represent a response to difficult social circumstances, it would be unwise to race to this conclusion and to dismiss other possibilities out of hand. Light-headedness means different things to different people: individuals with this symptom find their way into various clinics (neurology, cardiology, endocrinology, etc.) and a very wide range of diagnoses sometimes need to be considered. The combination of light-headedness with sweating and palpitations is a little more specific in that it suggests enhanced autonomic sympathetic activity (Table 8).

History of the presenting problem

The light-headedness, sweating and palpitations

It is important to ask the woman to explain as precisely as possible the nature of the episodes and to obtain a report from a witness if at all possible, since by the very nature of the problem the patient may not be able to give a lucid account. Ask both the patient and any witness about the following:

Table 8 Conditions presenting with light-headedness, sweating and palpitations.

Psychological/psychiatric	Anxiety state
'Toxic'	Excess use of stimulants, e.g. caffeine
	Alcohol withdrawal
	Drug withdrawal
Cardiovascular	Primary dysrhythmia
	Vasovagal
	Postural hypotension
Endocrine/metabolic	Menopausal vascular instability
	Hypoglycaemia
	Thyrotoxicosis
	Phaeochromocytoma

- When and how often do the episodes occur?
- What is she typically doing at the time?
- Are there any obvious precipitants?
- Is the onset sudden or gradual?
- What happens in an attack and how long does it last?
- Can she tap out how her heart beats at the time?
- Are some episodes worse than others?

Whilst answers to these questions may give a firm clue to one of the diagnoses listed in Table 8, it is also possible that the account given may broaden the differential diagnosis still further, and the full range of causes of presyncope, syncope or vertigo may need to be considered (see *Cardiology*, Sections 1.2 and 1.3; *Neurology*, Section 1.20).

Other issues

In addition to sweating and palpitations, are there any other autonomic symptoms, e.g. dry mouth, tremor, altered bowel habit? Consider the possibilities listed in Table 8 when talking with the patient.

- Anxiety/depression—does the patient experience pins and needles in the hands and feet, suggesting possible hyperventilation? Ask in detail about social circumstances, both at home and work, which seem likely to be relevant in this case from the information initially available. Does the woman have a long history of presenting with medically unexplained symptoms (see *Psychiatry*, Section 1.6)?
- Alcohol/drugs—how much alcohol does the patient drink? Does she take any drugs, prescribed or non-prescribed? These questions must be approached with tact and care (see *General clinical issues*, Section 2; *Gastroenterology and hepatology*, Sections 1.4 and 1.6). Is she 'addicted to coffee'?
- Cardiac dysrhythmias—both tachy- and bradydysrhythmias can be associated with light-headedness as a consequence of impaired cardiac output, and may be noted by the patient as 'palpitations'. Ask about shortness of breath and chest pain (see *Cardiology*, Sections 1.2 and 1.3).
- Endocrine/metabolic disorders—autonomic symptoms can be the presenting feature of both common (e.g. thyrotoxicosis) and uncommon (e.g. phaeochromocytoma) endocrine and metabolic conditions. Neuroglycopenia is a possible cause of 'light-headedness' and hypoglycaemia must be considered in this woman (Table 9). Ask about systemic symptoms, e.g. weight loss; if there is weight gain consider insulinoma.

Consider factitious hypoglycaemia

Factitious hypoglycaemia should be considered in those allied to the medical profession or, as in this case, where there is ease of access to insulin/oral hypoglycaemic agents.

Table 9 Causes of hypoglycaemia.

Category	Examples
Diabetes related	Inadequate carbohydrate intake, excessive exercise, pregnancy, inadvertent insulin/sulphony lurea overdose
Alcohol or drug induced	Salicylates, quinine, pentamidine
Tumour related	Insulinoma*, retroperitoneal sarcoma
Endocrine disorders	Hypopituitarism, Addison's disease, congenital adrenal hyperplasia
Hepatic dysfunction	Liver failure, inborn errors of metabolism, e.g. hereditary fructose intolerance
Reactive† (postprandial)	Idiopathic, postgastrectomy ('dumping syndrome')
Factitious	Sulphonylurea or insulin administration

*A history of fasting or exertion-related hypoglycaemia in an otherwise healthy adult should prompt consideration of insulinoma. Most cases are due to solitary benign tumours arising within the pancreas, although a small number have malignant potential and a few are seen in the context of the multiple endocrine neoplasia type 1 (MEN-1) syndrome (see Section 2.7, p. 115).

†Hypoglycaemia occurring within 5 h of ingestion of food. In most cases the diagnosis is one of exclusion, with hypoglycaemia documented during the presence of symptoms.

Examination

Light-headedness, sweating and palpitations

In any patient with episodic symptoms it is invaluable if they can be assessed during an attack: priorities (after ensuring airway, breathing and circulation) are to observe the general appearance, check the pulse, measure the blood pressure (BP), obtain an electocardiogram (ECG) rhythm strip and test for hypoglycaemia using a blood glucose test strip.

General

In a case such as this, your initial assessment is very important in gauging whether the symptoms have a psychological rather than physical origin—but beware of being blinded by your own prejudices! Always perform a full physical examination and, if relevant, assess psychological status.

Cardiovascular

Take careful note of the following:
• pulse—rate, rhythm and character
• BP—lying and standing
• heart sounds and murmurs—may indicate a structural basis for dysrhythmia.

Light-headedness, sweating and palpitations

• Hypoglycaemia—look for evidence of chronic liver disease, previous gastric surgery
• Hypopituitarism and Addison's disease
• Thyrotoxicosis—check for signs of thyrotoxicosis, e.g. tremor, warm peripheries, resting tachycardia, goitre and ophthalmopathy
• Phaeochromocytoma—is the patient hypertensive? Check for postural hypotension.

Approach to investigation and management

Investigations

Routine tests

Check full blood count (macrocytosis of chronic liver disease), electrolytes and renal function (Addison's disease), liver function (hepatic failure, metastases), fasting glucose, thyroid function tests (TFTs). Check chest radiograph (cardiac disease, metastases) and ECG (dysrhythmia).

Specific investigations

As dictated by clinical suspicion:
• cardiac disease—consider echocardiography and 24-h tape (see *Cardiology*, Section 2.2)
• liver disease/metastases—abdominal ultrasound; serological screen for intrinsic liver disorders
• Addison's disease—see Section 2.2.2, p. 60
• thyrotoxicosis—see Section 2.3.2, p. 70
• phaechromocytoma—see Section 2.2.5, p. 65.

HYPOGLYCAEMIA

If hypoglycaemia is shown to be the cause of symptoms, then in most instances the aetiology can be readily identified without recourse to further studies, e.g. diabetes related, liver disease. However, occasionally additional investigations are indicated.

Insulinoma

A supervised 72-h fast with regular measurements of glucose and insulin (every 6 h), and at any time when the patient is symptomatic, will unmask hypoglycaemia in most cases. Biochemical confirmation of hypoglycaemia (laboratory blood glucose <2.2 mmol/L) should be accompanied by demonstration of inappropriate hyperinsulinaemia and elevated C-peptide levels.

The tumour may be visible on ultrasound, CT (Fig. 2), MRI or coeliac axis angiography (Fig. 3), but up to one-third of cases are sufficiently small to evade detection. Accordingly, some centres advocate localization at surgery

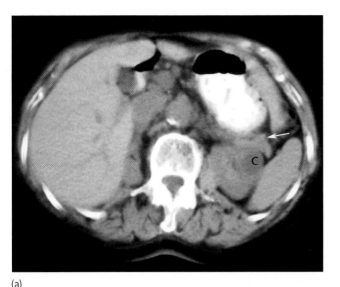

(a)

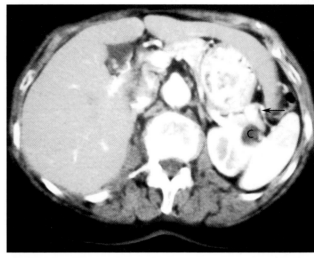

(b)

Fig. 2 Insulinoma. Pre- (a) and post-contrast (b) CT scans demonstrating an insulinoma (arrow) projecting anteriorly from the tail of the pancreas, in close proximity to an incidental left renal cyst (C).

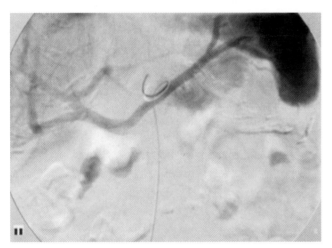

Fig. 3 Insulinoma tumour 'blush'. Digital subtraction angiogram of the splenic artery revealing the typical tumour 'blush' of an insulinoma within the tail of the pancreas.

by palpation under direct vision. Intraoperative ultrasound aids detection of tumours that are too small to feel.

Factitious hypoglycaemia
Exogenous insulin administration also causes hypoglycaemia with hyperinsulinaemia. However, because endogenous insulin secretion is suppressed, C-peptide levels are low.

By contrast, the surreptitious use of sulphonylureas (which enhance endogenous insulin secretion) gives rise to a biochemical profile similar to that seen with insulinoma. Plasma or urine sulphonylurea levels can be assayed to confirm suspicions.

Management

For Addison's disease, thyrotoxicosis and phaechromocytoma: see relevant sections of this module.

Hypoglycaemia

INSULINOMA

Surgical excision is the treatment of choice. Regular snacking will minimize the number of hypoglycaemic episodes prior to surgery. Diazoxide or somatostatin analogues, which inhibit insulin secretion, may be useful adjuncts in more refractory cases, or in those considered unfit for surgery.

REACTIVE HYPOGLYCAEMIA

Post-gastrectomy patients should be advised to eat little and often, avoiding rapidly absorbed carbohydrate. 'Idiopathic' (i.e. 'unexplained, but no sinister cause found') hypoglycaemia may respond to dietary manipulation with avoidance of refined carbohydrate and reassurance that there is no serious underlying disorder.

FACTITIOUS HYPOGLYCAEMIA

Confrontation is difficult and denial often occurs despite contradictory evidence. An underlying psychiatric condition is frequently present and appropriate referral is advisable.

 See *Emergency medicine*, Sections 1.17 and 1.26.
Karam JH. Hypoglycaemic disorders. In: Greenspan FS, Strewler GJ (eds) *Basic and Clinical Endocrinology*, 5th edn, pp. 664–679. Stanford: Appleton and Lange, 1997.

1.5 Crystals in the knee

Case history

A 40-year-old man with type 2 diabetes is referred from the Rheumatology ward. Aspiration of his acutely painful swollen right knee has revealed positively birefringent crystals of calcium pyrophosphate.

Clinical approach

Calcium pyrophosphate deposition disease ('pseudogout') (see *Rheumatology and clinical immunology*, Section 2.3.7), is the commonest cause of acute monoarthritis in the elderly. Its underlying cause (Table 10) should be actively sought, especially in younger patients such as this man. In this case, the history of type 2 diabetes at a young age is also unusual and should prompt specific consideration of a unifying diagnosis such as haemochromatosis.

The painful swollen joint

In the acutely painful swollen joint the immediate priority is to exclude infection—this can only be done by joint aspiration followed by microscopy and culture of joint fluid.

History of the presenting problem

The rheumatologists have already established the cause of the acute arthritis: for details on how to approach this presentation see *Rheumatology and clinical immunology*, Section 1.18.

It will be appropriate to ask about the history of type 2 diabetes and complications thereof (see Section 2.6, p. 100) but the main issue is to try to draw these things together. When taking the history pursue leads to possible diagnoses listed in Table 10:
• haemochromatosis—the only diagnosis likely to explain both diabetes and pseudogout. Excess iron deposition may lead to liver dysfunction (pruritus, easy bruising, etc.),

Table 10 Conditions associated with calcium pyrophosphate deposition disease.

Other joint disease	Osteoarthritis
	Gout
	Neuropathic joint
Metabolic disorders	Primary hyperparathyroidism
	Hypothyroidism
	Haemochromatosis
	Amyloidosis
	Hypomagnesaemia
	Wilson's disease

hypogonadism (diminished body hair, reduced libido and impotence), DM (polyuria, tiredness) and cardiac failure (dyspnoea, peripheral oedema, palpitations). Approximately 50% of cases are associated with arthritis, which is often the first sign of the condition. Involvement of the wrists and metacarpopharyngeal joints may mimic rheumatoid arthritis.

Also enquire about symptoms to support other possible causes of calcium pyrophosphate deposition disease, although none of these would be likely to account for the diabetes:
• primary hyperparathyroidism—ask about polyuria, polydipsia, constipation, previous urolithiasis (see Sections 1.2, p. 7 and 2.5.7, p. 95)
• hypothyroidism—weight gain, lethargy and cold intolerance would suggest undiagnosed hypothyroidism
• other joint disorders—enquire specifically about osteoarthritis and gout
• systemic disorders—which might predispose to amyloidosis
• excessive alcohol consumption—associated with gout and hypomagnesaemia.

Examination

Look for evidence of:
• skin pigmentation—slate grey in haemochromatosis
• complications of DM (see Section 2.6, p. 100)
• stigmata of chronic liver disease (*Gastroenterology and hepatology*, Sections 1.4, 1.6 and 2.10)
• hypogonadism (see Section 1.9, p. 21)
• hypothyroidism (see Section 2.3.1, p. 67)
• hyperparathyroidism (see Section 2.5.7, p. 95).

Cardiovascular

Is the heart normal? Take careful note of the pulse, BP, jugular venous pressure, apex beat, heart sounds, lung bases, and ankles, looking for signs of cardiomegaly/cardiac failure that can be a feature of haemochromatosis.

Abdomen

Examine specifically for hepatomegaly and check testicular size.

Musculoskeletal system

What is the pattern of joint involvement and the nature of any deformity?

Approach to investigation and management

Investigations

The most important investigation of any acute monoarthritis is joint aspiration and microscopy: this has already been undertaken to make the diagnosis of pseudogout. Further investigation is directed towards establishing the underlying cause.

Routine blood tests

These should include full blood count and inflammatory markers, fasting blood glucose and/or glycosylated haemoglobin (HbA_{1c}), liver function tests (haemochromatosis, Wilson's disease), calcium and phosphate (primary hyperparathyroidism), thyroid function tests (TFTs) and serum urate.

Radiology

Chondrocalcinosis may be evident in the affected joints (Fig. 4). Look for features suggestive of underlying osteoarthritis or gout (see *Rheumatology and clinical immunology*, Sections 2.3.2 and 2.3.6).

Tests for haemochromatosis

These are discussed in detail in Section 2.5.3, p. 89. In brief, consider:
• estimation of serum ferritin

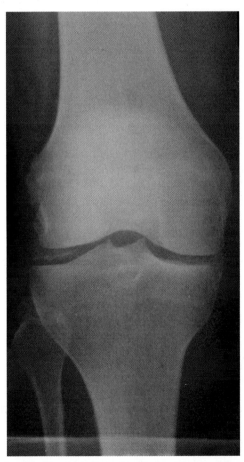

Fig. 4 Chondrocalcinosis. Radiograph of the knee showing linear calcification lying between and parallel to the articular surfaces.

• liver biopsy—demonstrates the presence and extent of hepatic iron deposition and excludes other coexistent pathology
• genetic screening—to identify mutations within the *HFE* gene
• gonadotrophins and testosterone—if haemochromatosis is confirmed, check luteinizing hormone (LH), follicle-stimulating hormone (FSH) and testosterone to exclude/confirm hypo- or hypergonadotrophic hypogonadism.

Ferritin is an acute phase reactant

Remember that in the setting of active inflammation the serum ferritin level is likely to be elevated. Therefore, when considering a diagnosis of haemochromatosis, a positive result should be confirmed once the C-reactive protein (CRP) has fallen to normal.

Management

For details of the management of acute monoarthritis, see *Rheumatology and clinical immunology*, Section 1.18.

The treatment of genetic haemochromatosis involves venesection to reduce iron overload (see Section 2.5.3, p. 89). Repeated venesection has little impact on arthritis once established, but it may prevent or delay its presentation if instituted early. Once a diagnosis of haemochromatosis is made, informed consent should be sought to allow screening of relatives.

Cox TM. Haemochromatosis. *Blood Reviews* 1990; 4: 75–87.
Griffiths WJH, Kelly AL, Cox TM. Inherited disorders of iron storage and transport. *Mol Med Today* 1999; 5: 431–438.

1.6 Hirsutism

Case history

A 33-year-old woman with long-standing irregular menses presents with gradually worsening hirsutism and weight gain. Both the beautician doing her electrolysis and a fellow 'Weight Watcher' have suggested that 'there might be something wrong with (her) glands', leading her to seek medical advice.

Clinical approach

Knowledge of the normal biology of hair growth is central to the understanding of hirsutism, a common disorder in endocrine clinics. Although most cases represent predominantly a cosmetic problem, occasionally hirsutism is a sign of serious underlying pathology (Table 11).

Table 11 Causes of hirsutism.

Common	Idiopathic
	Racial/familial
	PCOS
Less common	CAH
	Adrenal or ovarian androgen-secreting tumours
	Cushing's syndrome
	Hypothyroidism
	Other severe insulin resistance states
	Drugs, e.g. glucocorticoids, anabolic steroids

CAH, congenital adrenal hyperplasia; PCOS, polycystic ovarian syndrome.

Hair

- Hair can be classified as either vellus (soft, non-pigmented) or terminal (coarse, pigmented); prior to puberty most of the body is covered by vellus hair, notable exceptions being the scalp and eyebrows
- At puberty, under the influence of androgens, vellus hairs are transformed into terminal hairs. In females this process is limited mainly to the pubic and axillary regions
- The development in a female of terminal hairs in a male distribution (face, chest, back, lower abdomen and inner thighs) is referred to as hirsutism
- Enhanced conversion of testosterone to dihydrotestosterone (active metabolite), through increased 5α-reductase activity in skin, is believed to account for the majority of cases of idiopathic hirsutism
- Hirsutism should be distinguished from hypertrichosis, which is a generalized increase in vellus hair.

History of the presenting problem

Time course

It is important to determine the time course of the symptoms. The polycystic ovarian syndrome (PCOS) usually presents with gradual onset of hirsutism and weight gain on a background of long-standing oligomenorrhoea, typically dating back to puberty. By contrast, a more sudden onset of symptoms should prompt specific consideration of a virilizing adrenal or ovarian tumour.

Menstrual history and fertility

A detailed menstrual history is critical, including current or previous hormonal contraceptive use. It is important to know whether the patient is currently concerned about fertility, as this may influence the course of treatment you recommend.

Oral contraceptive pill

Remember that many women on the combined oral contraceptive pill regard their withdrawal bleeds as 'periods' and will truthfully say that they are regular.

Treatment of hirsutism

Ask about measures that the patient has used to control her hirsutism, e.g. depilatory creams, waxing, plucking, shaving, electrolysis.

Underlying disorders

Ask about symptoms of endocrine conditions that may be associated with hirsutism (Table 11).

Examination

On examination, you should note the following:
- body mass index (BMI) (women with PCOS may be overweight or obese, as is this woman)
- BP (elevated in some women with 'metabolic' PCOS)
- distribution and extent of hirsutism. Various scoring methods (e.g. the Ferriman–Gallwey system) have been devised to encourage more objective assessment of hirsutism
- signs of virilization (e.g. marked hirsutism, male pattern muscle development, clitoromegaly)—suggestive of adrenal or ovarian tumour
- abdominal or pelvic masses
- evidence of Cushing's syndrome or hypothyroidism.

Examination of the woman with hirsutism

Remember:
- the clinical picture may be modified by hair removal or make up
- there are significant variations in body hair in normal women from different ethnic backgrounds.

Approach to investigation and management

Investigation

Opinions differ as to the extent to which women with hirsutism should be investigated. A practical approach based on clinical findings is shown in Table 12. The features described in this case are suggestive of PCOS.

Investigation of hirsutism

- If suspected clinically, Cushing's syndrome and hypothyroidism require specific exclusion (see Section 2.1.1, p. 47 and 2.3.1, p. 67)
- Dehydroepiandrosterone sulphate (DHEAS), a pure adrenal androgen, is useful in differentiating adrenal from ovarian sources of hyperandrogenism
- If fertility is an issue, check day 21 progesterone (mid-luteal) to determine whether cycles are ovulatory.

Table 12 Strategy for the investigation of hirsutism.

Clinical presentation	Likely diagnosis	Investigation
Mild long-standing hirsutism with regular menses	Idiopathic	None (if the patient is concerned, LH, FSH and testosterone can be checked for reassurance)
Moderate hirsutism with long-standing irregular menses	Idiopathic, PCOS, CAH	LH, FSH, testosterone, DHEAS, 17α-hydroxyprogesterone (± ACTH stimulation), ± ovarian ultrasound
Severe hirsutism/rapid onset of symptoms/virilization/testosterone >6 nmol/L	CAH, adrenal/ovarian tumour	LH, FSH, testosterone, DHEAS, 17α-hydroxyprogesterone (± ACTH stimulation), ultrasound/CT/MRI of adrenals and ovaries

ACTH, adrenocorticotrophic hormone; CAH, congenital adrenal hyperplasia; CT, computed tomography; DHEAS, dehydroepiandrosterone sulphate; FSH, follicle-stimulating hormone; LH, luteinizing hormone; MRI, magnetic resonance imaging; PCOS, polycystic ovarian syndrome.

Management

This will clearly depend on the underlying diagnosis:
• Cushing's syndrome, congenital adrenal hyperplasia (CAH)—see Sections 2.1.1, p. 47 and 2.2.4, p. 63
• hypothyroidism—see Section 2.3.1, p. 67
• ovarian tumour—see *Oncology*, Section 2.5.
In the patient with PCOS, the following aspects are important.

Communication issues

Having excluded sinister underlying pathology, the patient should be reassured that, although there is a slight imbalance between the male and female hormones in her body, all women have some circulating male sex hormones and she is not being 'masculinized' in any way. Whilst it is important not to minimize symptoms that are troubling a patient, it may be appropriate to discuss the difference between the ideal woman portrayed by the media and the biological norm (in terms of body fat and hair distribution). Patients with relationship problems or eating disorders may receive additional benefit from liaison counselling or psychotherapy.

Weight loss

Weight loss ameliorates all of the symptoms of PCOS. Frequently, however, the patient has struggled to lose weight for many years, and may be unimpressed if, despite a hormonal imbalance being detected, there is nothing on offer other than a referral to the dietitian.

Hirsutism

Patients are usually experts on all forms of hair removal, having invested both time and money on a variety of cosmetic measures. Cyproterone acetate, an antiandrogen,

is effective but must not be used alone because of the potential risk to the unborn fetus. Simultaneous use of an oestrogen (e.g. ethinyloestradiol) provides effective contraception and, in addition, increases sex hormone binding globulin (SHBG) levels, thereby decreasing circulating free testosterone. Dianette®, a combined oral contraceptive pill that includes low-dose cyproterone acetate, is the formulation usually employed, frequently in combination with additional cyproterone to increase its antiandrogenic activity. spironolactone, which has antiandrogenic properties, is employed in countries where Dianette® is not available, e.g. in the USA.

Treatment of hirsutism

Whatever treatment is given, patients are often disappointed that 6 to 12 months may pass before any benefit is seen; it is important to emphasize this prior to initiating therapy.

Oligomenorrhoea/infertility

Normalization of the cycle can be achieved with a combined oral contraceptive pill, but ensure that you recommend a non-androgenic variety! Women with PCOS may not be in a relationship when they first seek medical advice, often attributing this to their hirsutism, however minimal this may seem to the objective observer. Whatever their current situation, it is important to point out that when fertility becomes an issue, they should seek medical help sooner rather than later. Women with PCOS often respond to clomiphene, although they may need specialist fertility treatment.

Other cardiovascular risk factors

Patients with the metabolic form of PCOS may be obese and have impaired glucose tolerance. Other cardiovascular risk factors (e.g. hypertension, smoking, lipid profile) should be reviewed and treated as necessary (see Section 1.17, p. 38).

> Carmina E, Lobo RA. Polycystic ovary syndrome: arguably the most common endocrinopathy is associated with significant morbidity in women. *J Clin Endocrinol Metab* 1999; 84: 1897–1899.
>
> Conn JJ, Jacobs HS. The clinical management of hirsutism. *Eur J Endocrinol* 1997; 136: 339–348.
>
> Rittmaster RS. Hirsutism. *Lancet* 1997; 349: 191–195.

1.7 Post-pill amenorrhoea

Case history

A 28-year-old woman is referred for investigation of 'post-pill amenorrhoea'. Her menstrual history is unremarkable, with menarche at 13 years of age and a regular cycle prior to going onto the oral contraceptive pill aged 18. However, her periods have not returned since coming off the pill 2 years ago and she is now keen to start a family.

Clinical approach

The presentation is one of secondary amenorrhoea with infertility. 'Post-pill amenorrhoea' is not a diagnosis in itself: some other pathology must be implicated.

History of the presenting problem

When taking the history, think about the following possible diagnoses as you do so:
• pregnancy—even allowing for the duration of amenorrhoea, pregnancy must be excluded in all cases
• exercise/dieting/stress—excessive exercise, weight loss or psychological stress can suppress the activity of the gonadotrophin-releasing hormone (GnRH) pulse generator. Patients may be evasive in their answers to questions concerning these issues
• pituitary disease—secondary amenorrhoea can reflect direct damage to the gonadotrophs (e.g. pituitary adenoma, infarction) or hyperprolactinaemia (which disrupts GnRH neuronal activity). Enquire about galactorrhoea and other symptoms of pituitary disease (see Section 2.1, p. 47)
• premature ovarian failure (POF)—most commonly autoimmune in origin and characterized by hypergonadotrophic hypogonadism. Ask about menopausal symptoms, e.g. hot flushes, dyspareunia and check for a family history of early menopause
• adrenal or ovarian tumours—enquire about hirsutism and

virilizing features (see Section 1.6, p. 16). Given the preceding menstrual history, both the PCOS and CAH are less likely.

Examination

A full physical examination should be performed, paying particular attention to:
• BMI (extremes may be associated with oligomenorrhoea or amenorrhoea)
• hirsutism, acne or virilization
• visual fields (looking for bitemporal hemianopia)
• galactorrhoea (indicating hyperprolactinaemia).

Approach to investigation and management

Investigations

Pregnancy test

However unlikely it may seem, it is important to exclude pregnancy before embarking on further investigations. Routine blood tests will often have been checked before the patient is referred (e.g. full blood count, urea and electrolytes, calcium, liver biochemistry and thyroid function).

Specific endocrine assessment

Check:
• LH, FSH and oestradiol (E_2) (to distinguish hypo- and hypergonadotrophic hypogonadism)
• prolactin (elevated in prolactinoma or with stalk disconnection)
• testosterone and DHEAS (to exclude ovarian or adrenal tumour)
Further investigations will be guided by the clinical features and initial biochemical screen:
• hyperprolactinaemia and hypopituitarism—see Section 2.1.3, p. 51 and 2.1.7, p. 57
• POF—see Section 2.4.1, p. 76.

Management

This will clearly depend on the diagnosis:
• pregnancy—it is rare for pregnancy to present to an endocrine clinic: the chances are that you won't be the only surprised person in the room!
• excessive exercise/weight loss/stress—explain the physiological basis for the amenorrhoea and encourage moderation. Psychological/psychiatric input may be required
• POF—see Section 2.4.1, p. 76
• hyperprolactinaemia—see Section 2.1.3, p. 51
• non-functioning pituitary tumour—see Section 2.1.4, p. 54.

Education of the patient with a pituitary tumour

Patients with pituitary problems need to understand a little anatomy and physiology, otherwise their disease, its monitoring and treatment can seem very mysterious. They will often have their own ideas about 'brain tumours': it is important to find out what these are and if necessary provide reassurance that their type of tumour will not spread elsewhere in the body, and will not need treatment that results in baldness, etc. Patient information leaflets produced by the Pituitary Foundation are a useful aid.

Education of the patient with a pituitary tumour

Patients with microprolactinomas who are not trying to conceive need to be aware of the importance of complying with treatment to prevent osteoporosis: many women are quite happy not having periods when they know there is 'nothing to worry about'. If they find the side-effects of bromocriptine upsetting, oestrogen replacement therapy is a good alternative.

Baird DT. Amenorrhoea. *Lancet* 1997; 350: 275–279.
Colao A, Lombardi G. Growth hormone and prolactin excess. *Lancet* 1998; 352: 1455–1461.
Levy A, Lightman SL. Diagnosis and management of pituitary tumours. *BMJ* 1994; 308: 1087–1091.
Schlechte JA. Clinical impact of hyperprolactinaemia. *Baillière's Clin Endocrinol Metab* 1995; 9: 359–366.

1.8 Short girl with no periods

Case history

A young woman presents at 15 years of age because her menstrual periods have not started. She is in good health, but tells you with some feeling that she is 'the shortest person' in her class at school. On examination, it is clear that she has not yet developed any secondary sexual characteristics.

Clinical approach

'Delayed growth and puberty' are often linked presentations (see Section 2.4.5, p. 82). Investigations should be initiated if there are no secondary sexual characteristics by 14 years of age in girls and $14\frac{1}{2}$ years of age in boys.

History of the presenting problem

During the initial assessment it is useful to consider the following points.
• Is data showing the time course of growth failure available, e.g. child health records which include growth charts (Fig. 5)? Enquire about birth weight and problems at delivery since low birth weight is associated with short stature.

• Does she have a history of other chronic illness, e.g. asthma, cystic fibrosis, Crohn's disease, CRF? Any of these can lead to short stature.
• Is there a family history of short stature or delayed puberty?
• What are her eating habits? Both nutritional deficiency and disorders such as anorexia nervosa are associated with short stature.
• What are her social circumstances? Emotional stress can have adverse effects on growth.

Examination

A thorough examination is necessary, looking for signs of systemic illness, e.g. chronic lung disease. You should also make a note of:
• height, weight and arm span: this will help to determine whether growth failure is uniformly distributed
• pubertal stage (see Section 1.9, p. 23)
• features suggesting a specific diagnosis, e.g. Turner's syndrome or other genetic, endocrine or dysmorphic syndromes, e.g. achondroplasia.

Turner's syndrome

Look for the classical stigmata: webbed neck, low hairline, widely spaced nipples, cubitus valgus (Fig. 6). Remember, however, that the clinical features may be attenuated if there is only partial X chromosome deletion or alternatively mosaicism (see *Genetics and molecular medicine*, Section 4).

Approach to investigation and management

Investigations

There are a number of chronic diseases that can be easily diagnosed and are worth screening for on a fairly universal basis. Recommended blood tests, imaging and further investigations are detailed in Section 2.4.5 (p. 82).

Turner's syndrome

Patients with classical Turner's syndrome (as in this case) usually exhibit:
• low/undetectable E_2 with high levels of LH and FSH (hypergonadotrophic hypogonadism)
• 45 XO karyotype.
Further investigations in confirmed cases of Turner's syndrome are discussed below.

Management

General guidelines for the management of children with delayed puberty and/or short stature are outlined in Section 2.4.5, p. 82.

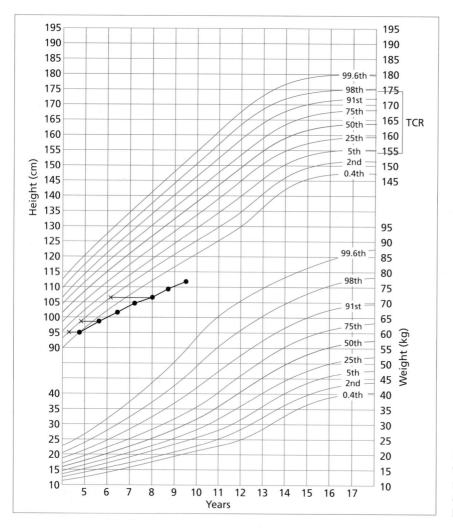

Fig. 5 Growth chart from a young girl with Turner's syndrome. The dots denote measurements plotted according to chronological age, whilst the crosses refer to bone age. TCR, target centile range.

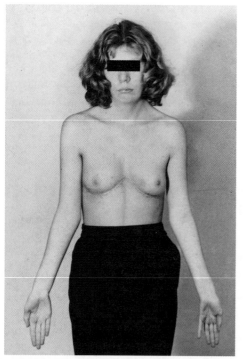

Fig. 6 Turner's syndrome. Note the webbed neck and wide carrying angle, which are typical of classical Turner's syndrome. In addition, there is a visible thoracotomy scar from a previous atrial septal defect repair.

Turner's syndrome

There are many issues, both physical and psychological, that need to be addressed in the management of women with Turner's syndrome.

HORMONE REPLACEMENT THERAPY

A natural oestrogen will promote the development of secondary sexual characteristics. Treatment should be started at a low dose and gradually increased. After 1 or 2 years, maintenance treatment with cyclical oestrogen and progestogen therapy can be started.

 Treatment of Turner's syndrome

The timing of oestrogen replacement is critical. It is often delayed to maximize final height, especially if growth hormone (GH) therapy is used (see below).

OSTEOPOROSIS

Women with Turner's syndrome are at an increased risk of developing osteoporosis. In addition to oestrogen replacement therapy their diet should be checked to ensure an adequate supply of calcium, and regular weight-bearing exercise encouraged.

ISCHAEMIC HEART DISEASE

A three-fold excess mortality from ischaemic heart disease (IHD) probably reflects an increased incidence of insulin resistance/type 2 diabetes and hypertension. Both of these conditions should therefore be sought and treated, and the benefits of hormone replacement therapy (HRT), weight control and exercise reiterated.

STRUCTURAL CARDIAC AND RENAL ABNORMALITIES

Echocardiography and renal ultrasonography may reveal structural abnormalities. In addition to any specific management that might be indicated, prompt treatment of urinary tract infections and antibiotic prophylaxis against infective endocarditis should be considered. A bicuspid aortic valve is the commonest cardiac abnormality and may be associated with progressive aortic root dilatation. Good BP control is essential.

HYPOTHYROIDISM

Turner's syndrome is associated with a high incidence of primary autoimmune hypothyroidism (Hashimoto's thyroiditis): regular TFTs are recommended.

CRYPTIC Y CHROMOSOME MATERIAL

Karyotyping may reveal cryptic Y chromosome material (45 XO/46 XY). This predisposes to gonadoblastoma and is an indication for prophylactic gonadectomy (or close observation).

FERTILITY

Between 2 and 5% of women with Turner's syndrome have spontaneous menstrual periods, although only 0.5% have ovulatory cycles and an early menopause is likely. Contraceptive advice and genetic counselling are important in this subgroup, since there is an approximately 30% risk that their offspring will have a congenital anomaly. For the majority of cases, however, specialist fertility input is required if they wish to conceive by *in-vitro* fertilization (IVF) or gamete intra fallopian transfer (GIFT) using a donor ovum. Prepregnancy cardiovascular and renal screening is imperative.

INTELLIGENCE

Intelligence is generally normal, although hand–eye coordination, social and visuospatial skills may be impaired.

SHORT STATURE

Although children with Turner's syndrome are not GH deficient, treatment with recombinant human GH (either alone or in combination with anabolic agents such as oxandrolone) may increase their final adult height.

Turner's syndrome—ethical issues and communication

There are many important psychological issues to consider in caring for women with Turner's syndrome. Most importantly, to quote from literature produced by the Turner's Society, 'women with Turner's syndrome should have no doubt of their femininity: physically, behaviourally and sexually'. A number of the management issues outlined above may be self-evident to a physician, but confusing to the patient unless fully explained:
- the need for gonadectomy if there is cryptic Y material, even though the ovaries are non-functioning
- the need for 'periods' (rather than unopposed oestrogen therapy)
- that 'periods' are actually withdrawal bleeds and do not represent restored fertility
- why the patient is prescribed the low-dose combined oral contraceptive pill even though she is infertile.

Alabnese A, Stanhope R. Investigation of delayed puberty. *Clin Endocrinol* 1995; 43: 105–110.
Saenger P. Turner's syndrome. *N Engl J Med* 1996; 335: 1749–1754.
Stanhope R, Jacobs H, Slater C. *The Turner Woman: A Patient's Guide*, Series 9. The Child Growth Foundation/The Turner Society.

1.9 Young man who has 'not developed'

Case history

An 18-year-old man is referred by his GP who had incidentally noted him to be hypogonadal during a recent consultation. He has no past medical history of note.

Clinical approach

Table 13 outlines the major groups of disorders associated with male hypogonadism, a term that denotes deficiency of both testosterone secretion (from Leydig cells) and sperm production (by the seminiferous tubules).

> **Male hypogonadism**
>
> • Klinefelter's syndrome—congenital disorder associated with an abnormal karyotype (47XXY). Characterized by small firm testes, small phallus, eunuchoid proportions and gynaecomastia. Azoospermia reflects seminiferous tubule dysgenesis. Testosterone production is variable, leading to differing degrees of sexual development.
> • Kallmann's syndrome—congenital disorder characterized by isolated gonadotrophin deficiency and hypoplasia of the olfactory lobes, leading to anosmia. A number of cases have deletions of the *KAL* gene on the X chromosome. Undescended testes and gynaecomastia are recognized associations.

Table 13 Aetiology of male hypogonadism.

Primary hypogonadism (i.e. testicular dysfunction)	Idiopathic
	Post chemotherapy, viral orchitis or trauma
	Klinefelter's syndrome
	Systemic disorders, e.g. renal failure, haemochromatosis, myotonic dystrophy
Secondary hypogonadism (i.e. hypothalamic/pituitary in origin)	Constitutional delayed puberty
	Hyperprolactinaemia
	Pituitary tumour/infiltration/surgery/ radiotherapy
	Kallmann's syndrome
	Idiopathic hypogonadotrophic hypogonadism

History of the presenting problem

Androgen status

Ask about:
• frequency of shaving and beard growth
• axillary and pubic hair development
• deepening of the voice
• libido, erectile function (and where appropriate fertility).

Hypogonadotrophic hypogonadism

Enquire about:
• problems with sense of smell (hyposmia or anosmia in Kallmann's syndrome)
• features suggesting other pituitary hormone deficiencies (Section 2.1.7, p. 57)
• headaches/visual problems (pituitary space-occupying lesion)
• galactorrhoea (hyperprolactinaemia).

Hypergonadotrophic hypogonadism

Ask about:
• testicular trauma or bilateral orchitis in the past
• gynaecomastia (Klinefelter's syndrome).

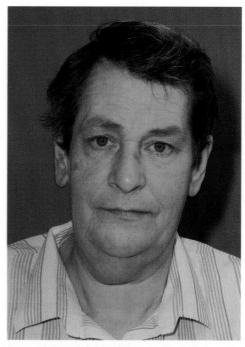

Fig. 7 Hypogonadal male. Note the absence of facial hair and fine wrinkles around the corners of the eyes and mouth.

Relevant past history

Although in this particular case there was no past medical history of note, in general it is important to enquire about previous illnesses. A family history of delayed puberty may be relevant in Kallmann's syndrome and in simple constitutional delayed puberty.

Examination

General

Long-standing hypogonadism often gives rise to a distinctive facial appearance, especially in older men in whom the poverty of facial hair and lack of temporal recession is most noticeable (Fig. 7). Also check in particular for:
• an impaired sense of smell (Kallmann's syndrome)
• eunuchoid habitus (i.e. span greater than height and heel to pubis distance greater than pubis to crown), which is common in those in whom hypogonadism precedes puberty, e.g. Klinefelter's syndrome
• gynaecomastia—indicates a decrease in the androgen : oestrogen ratio
• galactorrhoea (hyperprolactinaemia).

Assess pubertal development

The Tanner Staging System (Tables 14 and 15) allows for an objective assessment of sexual maturity. In recognition of the differing actions of adrenal androgens and gonadal steroids, it distinguishes between genital and pubic hair development in boys and breast and pubic hair development in girls.

Table 14 Tanner pubertal stages in boys.

Area of development	Stage	Description
Genital	1	Pre-adolescent: testes, scrotum and penis are of about the same size and proportion as in early childhood
	2	Enlargement of scrotum and testes. Skin of scrotum reddens and changes in texture. Little or no enlargement of the penis at this stage
	3	Enlargement of the penis, which occurs at first mainly in length. Further growth of testes and scrotum
	4	Increased size of penis with growth in breadth and development of glans. Testes and scrotum larger; scrotal skin darkened
	5	Genitalia adult in size and shape
Pubic hair	1	Pre-adolescent: the vellus over the pubes is not further developed than that over the abdominal wall, i.e. no pubic hair
	2	Sparse growth of long, slightly pigmented downy hair, straight or slightly curled, chiefly at the base of the penis
	3	Considerably darker, coarser and more curled. The hair spreads sparsely laterally
	4	Hair now adult in type, but the area covered is still considerably smaller than in the adult. No spread to medial surface of the thighs
	5	Adult in quantity and type

Table 15 Tanner pubertal stages in girls.

Area of development	Stage	Description
Breast	1	Pre-adolescent: elevation of papilla only
	2	Breast bud stage: elevation of breast and papilla as small mound. Enlargement of areolar diameter
	3	Further enlargement and elevation of breast and areola, with no separation of their contours
	4	Projection of areola and papilla to form a secondary mound above the level of the breast
	5	Mature stage: projection of papilla only, due to recession of the areola to the general contour of the breast
Pubic hair	1	Pre-adolescent: the vellus over the pubes is not further developed than that over the abdominal wall, i.e. no pubic hair
	2	Sparse growth of long, slightly pigmented downy hair, straight or slightly curled, chiefly along labia
	3	Considerably darker, coarser and more curled. The hair spreads sparsely over the junction of the pubes
	4	Hair now adult in type, but the area covered is still considerably smaller than in the adult. No spread to medial surface of the thighs
	5	Adult in quantity and type

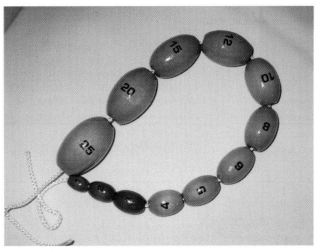

Fig. 8 Prader orchidometer.

The presence of bilateral descended testes should be confirmed by palpation and testicular volume assessed with an orchidometer (Fig. 8).

The patient with hypogonadism

Cryptorchidism (unilateral or bilateral absence of the testes from the scrotum) is an important clinical finding since it indicates a significant risk of malignant transformation in the affected gonad(s) and further investigation is mandatory (see below).

Assess pituitary status

Check for features suggestive of a pituitary tumour, e.g. bitemporal hemianopia, hypopituitarism.

Approach to investigation and management

Investigations

Routine blood tests

Unless the clinical features suggest a specific underlying disorder, some simple screening tests should be performed including: full blood count (anaemia), urea and electrolytes (chronic renal impairment), fasting glucose, thyroid function, prolactin, liver biochemistry and serum ferritin (haemochromatosis).

Luteinizing hormone, follicle-stimulating hormone and testosterone

A low testosterone level confirms hypogonadism. Measurement of LH and FSH allows distinction between hypogonadotrophic and hypergonadotrophic hypogonadism, although remember that the former may simply indicate constitutional delay.

Specific investigations

These will be guided by your clinical impression and preliminary screening tests, but may include:

- karyotype analysis—to exclude Klinefelter's syndrome
- assessment of pituitary function/MRI pituitary fossa—in cases of secondary hypogonadism/hyperprolactinaemia (see Sections 2.1.7, p. 57 and 2.1.3, p. 51)
- ultrasound of the testes—the clinical finding of cryptorchidism must be investigated further to try and identify the site of the undescended/maldescended tissue
- semen analysis—including assessment of number, morphology and motility
- human chorionic gonadotrophin (hCG) stimulation—hCG is able to mimic the ability of LH to stimulate testosterone synthesis and secretion, and therefore may help to differentiate primary and secondary gonadal failure
- bone densitometry (dual energy X-ray absorptiometry [DEXA])-testosterone is required for maintenance of normal bone mineral density (BMD) in men. Bone densitometry may help to identify those at significant risk of fracture, and is particularly useful in older men who decline testosterone replacement, when alternative prophylaxis should be offered, e.g. with a bisphosphonate.

Management

General

The general principles governing management of the hypogonadal male include:

- patient and sympathetic explanation
- treatment of any underlying disorder
- replacement of hormone deficiency
- referral for specialist fertility advice if appropriate.

Various preparations of testosterone replacement are available and are discussed in more detail in Section 2.1.7, p. 57.

 Belchetz P. Male hypogonadism. In: Grossman A (ed.). *Clinical Endocrinolgy*, 2nd edn, pp. 666–686. Oxford: Blackwell Science, 1998.

1.10 Depression and diabetes

Case history

A normally active 72-year-old widow is taken to her family doctor by her caring relatives who are concerned about her mental state: they fear she is depressed. Her past medical history is unremarkable, although she is

Table 16 Physical illnesses with depression as a common presenting feature.

Type of problem	Example	
'Obvious'	Any condition causing severe physical debility	Malignancy 'Systemic illness', e.g. advanced cardiac/respiratory failure or chronic renal failure (dialysis) Parkinson's disease
	Any condition causing chronic pain	'Arthritis/rheumatism' Refractory headache Post-herpetic neuralgia
'More subtle'	Endocrine	Hypothyroidism Hyperparathyroidism Cushing's syndrome
	Neurological	Dementia

overweight and routine urinalysis by the GP has revealed glycosuria.

Clinical approach

Depression is very common. There may be several contributing factors, e.g. social isolation, neglect, bereavement, poverty and chronic health problems: all are major risk factors that should be sought in the history. Remember, however, that depression can be a manifestation of many physical illnesses, particularly in the elderly, as shown in Table 16.

History of the presenting problem

Since the presenting problem is, or might be, depression enquire about physical and psychological features of depressive illness (see *Psychiatry*, Sections 2.6 and 2.11).

However, since physical illness can masquerade as depression, a full medical history and systems enquiry is required to look for evidence of any of the conditions listed in Table 16. This will clearly involve exploration of matters related to diabetes given that she has been found to have glycosuria. Has this been documented previously? Have there been symptoms of thirst and polyuria (see Section 2.6, p. 101)? Also think about the following as you take the history:

- Cushing's syndrome/pseudo-Cushing's syndrome—type 2 diabetes is common in the elderly obese population, but when associated with mood change should prompt consideration of Cushing's syndrome. Enquire about symptoms of glucocorticoid excess, e.g. easy bruising, difficulty climbing stairs (see Section 2.1.1, p. 47). Check for an obvious cause, e.g. exogenous steroid usage, and enquire about alcohol consumption. Remember depression and excessive alcohol intake can result in pseudo-Cushing's syndrome (see Section 2.1.1, p. 48). Care and tact will be required to elicit this history (see *General clinical issues*, Section 2)

• hypothyroidism—mood change and weight gain are recognized features of hypothyroidism (see Section 2.3.1, p. 68)
• hypercalcaemia—remember 'bones, stones, abdominal groans and psychic moans'
• dementia, e.g. Alzheimer's disease; multi-infarct dementia—may be mistaken for a depressive illness in the early stages (see *Medicine for the elderly*, Section 2.7).

Enquire about home circumstances and social support available.

Examination

General

Remember the psychiatric assessment: appearance, general behaviour, speech, thought, abnormal beliefs and interpretation of events (see *Psychiatry*, Sections 1.6 and 2.5).

A thorough physical examination of all systems is required, but with particular attention to the following possibilities:
• DM—see Section 2.6, p. 100
• Cushing's syndrome—does the patient exhibit centripetal obesity? Check for bruises, purple striae and proximal myopathy (see Section 2.1.1, p. 47)
• hypothyroidism—see Section 2.3.1, p. 67
• hypercalcaemia—unlikely to produce any physical signs, but is there band keratopathy
• Parkinson's disease—check for the classic triad of resting tremor, bradykinesia and cogwheel rigidity (see *Neurology*, Sections 1.3 and 2.3)
• dementia—assess the mental state, e.g. mini mental state examination (see *Medicine for the elderly*, Section 3.2).

Approach to investigation and management

Investigations

Initial tests

• Check full blood count (normochromic normocytic anaemia of systemic disease), urea and electrolytes (renal impairment; hypokalaemia—ectopic Cushing's syndrome), liver chemistry and calcium (hypercalcaemia, metastases), fasting glucose and thyroid function tests (TFTs). Consider performing a full dementia screen (see *Medicine for the elderly*, Sections 1.2 and 2.7)
• Check chest radiograph to look for evidence of bronchial neoplasia/lymphadenopathy
• Check ECG.

Specific investigations and management

These will be directed by the suspicions raised on history, examination and initial testing:
• DM (see Section 2.6, p. 100)
• Cushing's syndrome (see Section 2.1.1, p. 47) (the actual diagnosis in this case)
• hypothyroidism (see Section 2.3.1, p. 67)
• hypercalcaemia (see Section 2.5.8, p. 97)
• Parkinson's disease (see *Neurology*, Section 2.3)
• dementia (see *Medicine for the elderly*, Section 2.7).

1.11 Acromegaly

Case history

A 37-year-old man is referred for further investigation by an anaesthetic colleague who has diagnosed acromegaly during preoperative assessment for carpal tunnel decompression. A random GH level has been checked and found to be high.

Clinical approach

Clearly a clinical suspicion of acromegaly in a patient awaiting carpal tunnel decompression must be taken seriously. However, do not assume that the diagnosis has been confirmed on the basis of a single 'high' GH measurement.

Secretion of growth hormone

Normal GH secretion is pulsatile. Therefore random GH levels do not reliably discriminate between normal subjects and those with acromegaly unless markedly elevated.

History of the presenting problem

Local tumour expansion

Ask about:
• headaches
• visual disturbance.

Growth hormone excess

Consider the following:
• Have there been any changes in ring, shoe or hat size?
• Has there been any alteration/coarsening of features?
• Does he snore?
• Does he sweat excessively?

- Ask about arthritis and arthralgia.
- Check for symptoms of cardiac failure.
- DM—GH antagonizes the action of insulin, hence enquire about polyuria, polydipsia, tiredness and lethargy.
- Hypertension—has his BP ever been measured? Hypertension is a major factor contributing to the excess morbidity and mortality seen in untreated acromegaly.

Pituitary dysfunction

Enquire about reduced libido and difficulties achieving/maintaining an erection (hypogonadism), tiredness and dizziness (adrenocorticotrophic hormone [ACTH] deficiency), weight gain and lethargy (hypothyroidism), galactorrhoea (hyperprolactinaemia).

Relevant past history

Remember that acromegaly can arise in the setting of multiple endocrine neoplasia type 1 (MEN-1) (see Section 2.7, p. 115). Check for a history of hypercalcaemia and ask about relatives with similar problems.

Examination

Acromegaly

A picture is worth a thousand words. Ask the patient to bring along old photographs that may allow you to determine the approximate date of onset of the condition.

Look for the typical facial appearance: greasy skin, prominent supraorbital ridges, broad nose, thick lips, large tongue (Fig. 9). Check for evidence of proganthism and a goitre. Then carefully examine the following:
- hands—look for 'spade-like' hands (Fig. 10) with greasy skin and excessive sweating; also for signs of carpal tunnel syndrome (clearly present in this case)
- eyes—assess visual acuity, examine visual fields to confrontation (looking for evidence of a bitemporal hemianopia) and test for ophthalmoplegia (reflecting lateral extension of the pituitary tumour)
- cardiovascular system—record the BP and look for signs of heart failure
- signs of hypopituitarism—look for evidence of pituitary hormone deficiencies (see Section 2.1.7, p. 57) and hyperprolactinaemia (see Section 2.1.3, p. 52).

Approach to investigation and management

These are covered in detail in Section 2.1.2 (p. 50) and Section 3.2.3 (p. 122). In brief:
- the oral glucose tolerance test (OGTT) remains the

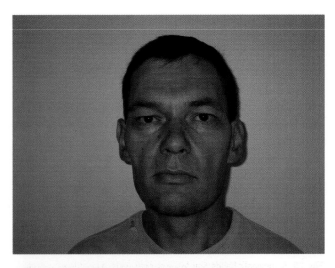

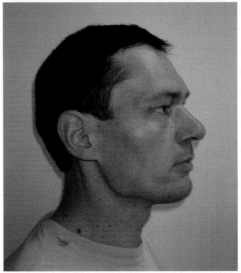

Fig. 9 Acromegalic facies, showing the typical coarse facial features with prominent supraorbital ridges, prognathism and multiple skin tags.

'gold standard' investigation for confirming/excluding acromegaly
- insulin-like growth factor (IGF-I) levels are typically elevated above the age-related normal range and can be used to monitor the effectiveness of treatment
- MRI of the pituitary fossa distinguishes macro- from microadenomas. It is also important postoperatively to guide the choice of adjunctive treatment in cases where transsphenoidal surgery is not curative.

 Colao A, Lombardi G. Growth hormone and prolactin excess. *Lancet* 1998; 352: 1455–1461.

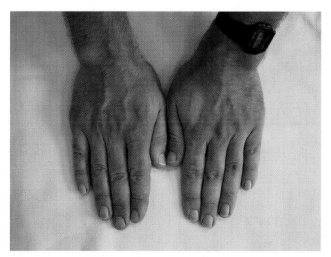

Fig. 10 Acromegalic hands. Soft tissue growth leads to enlargement of the hands and thickening of the digits, which take on a 'spade-like' appearance.

1.12 Postpartum amenorrhoea

Case history

A 27-year-old woman is referred for investigation of secondary amenorrhoea, which dates back to the birth of her first child 8 months earlier. She also reports increasing tiredness and lethargy.

Clinical approach

Although any of the recognized causes of secondary amenorrhoea (see Section 2.4.1, p. 77) can present for the first time in the postpartum period, two conditions merit special consideration:
• Sheehan's syndrome—postpartum pituitary infarction
• lymphocytic hypophysitis—an autoimmune disorder characterized by lymphocytic infiltration of the pituitary gland, typically presenting in the third trimester or postpartum period with a pituitary mass and/or hypopituitarism.

History of the presenting problem

Ascertain details of the patient's previous menstrual history, including age at menarche, regularity of cycle, oral contraceptive use, previous spells of oligomenorrhoea/amenorrhoea and problems with fertility.

Could physiological causes be responsible? Is she continuing to lactate, or is there a possibility of a further pregnancy? Then consider the following.

Hypothalamic–pituitary disorders

Clues to the presence of a hypothalamic–pituitary disorder might be:

• headaches or visual disturbances (local tumour expansion) or galactorrhoea (hyperprolactinaemia)
• symptoms suggestive of pituitary hormone deficiency. When did the tiredness and lethargy first become apparent? Ask about postural dizziness, loss of pubic and axillary hair and lack of libido. Is there a history of polyuria/polydipsia following delivery? Diabetes insipidus (DI) has been reported with both Sheehan's syndrome and lymphocytic hypophysitis
• problems during or after delivery, especially intrapartum or postpartum haemorrhage (Sheehan's syndrome). Obtain and review the obstetric records
• did she choose to breastfeed her first child, and if so was this successful? Failure of lactation may indicate Sheehan's syndrome or lymphocytic hypophysitis.

Other conditions

Consider PCOS, especially if there is a history of preceding oligomenorrhoea/amenorrhoea and difficulty with conception. Also think about ovarian/adrenal tumours: these are much less likely, but a history of recent-onset hirsutism/virilization should raise concerns (see Section 1.6, p. 15).

Relevant past history

A history of other organ-specific autoimmune disorders, e.g. Hashimoto's disease, Addison's disease, is more common in lymphocytic hypophysitis.

Ask about recent weight loss, dietary habits and social circumstances. Juggling the demands of a newborn baby with a return to work can be particularly stressful and could cause amenorrhoea!

Examination

A full physical examination is required, taking particular note of the following:
• weight, height and calculate BMI
• evidence of gonadotrophin deficiency—loss of pubic and axillary hair, breast tissue atrophy
• other features of hypopituitarism—physical signs may include soft, fine and wrinkled skin; pallor; postural hypotension
• possibility of pituitary mass lesions (e.g. macroadenoma, lymphocytic hypophysitis)—examine visual fields looking for evidence of a bitemporal hemianopia; exclude cranial nerve (III, IV, V, VI) involvement
• could there be hyperprolactinaemia? Examine for galactorrhoea
• might there be PCOS or an adrenal/ovarian tumour? Check for evidence of hirsutism or virilization (see Section 1.6, p. 15).

Approach to investigations and management

Investigations

A strategy for the investigation of amenorrhoea is set out in Section 2.4.1, p. 76. Important points relating to the investigation of Sheehan's syndrome and lymphocytic hypophysitis are:

• DI—paired serum and urine osmolalities may confirm your clinical suspicions. More formal assessment with a water deprivation test should be deferred until thyroid and adrenal insufficiency have been excluded or adequately treated

• pituitary MRI/CT—lymphocytic hypophysitis gives rise to a distinctive appearance on MRI/CT examination (Fig. 11). Symmetrical enlargement of the gland is typically accompanied by a dome-shaped suprasellar extension which often abuts/compresses the optic chiasm

• pituitary biopsy/decompression controversy remains as to whether a clinical diagnosis of lymphocytic hypophysitis should be confirmed by pituitary biopsy to avoid the possibility of misdiagnosing a non-functioning pituitary adenoma.

Management

> **Postpartum amenorrhoea**
>
> • Adrenal insufficiency must be excluded/corrected before thyroid replacement is commenced (Section 2.1.7, p. 57)
> • Sight-threatening pituitary enlargement in lymphocytic hypophysitis should be referred for urgent surgical decompression.

Management of specific hypothalamic/pituitary disorders is given in Section 2.1, p. 47 and for causes of amenorrhoea in Section 2.4.1, p. 76. Appropriate hormone replacement therapy is the mainstay of treatment for both Sheehan's syndrome and lymphocytic hypophysitis. High dose corticosteroids may be used in the latter to 'dampen down' the inflammatory process.

Ezzat S, Josse RG. Autoimmune hypophysitis. *Trends Endocrinol Metab* 1997; 8(2):74–80.
Patel MC, Guneratne N, Haq N, West TET, Weetman AP, Clayton RW. Peripartum hypopituitarism and lymphocytic hypophysitis. *Q J Med* 1995; 88: 571–580.

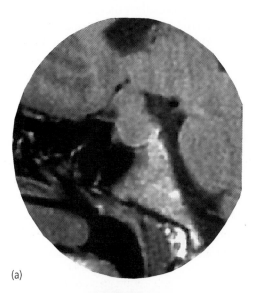

(a)

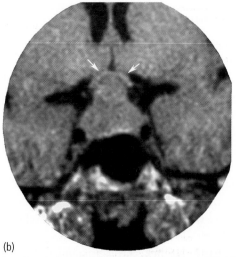

(b)

Fig. 11 Lymphocytic hypophysitis. Sagittal (a) and coronal (b) MRI scans demonstrating symmetrical pituitary enlargement with suprasellar extension in a young pregnant woman, who presented with a bitemporal field defect at 36 weeks' gestation. The optic chiasm is visible, compressed against the top of the pituitary swelling (arrows).

1.13 Weight loss

Case history

A 20-year-old hairdresser has lost more than 2 stones in weight within the last 3 months. She feels tired most of the time and keeps getting into arguments at work.

Clinical approach

Weight loss is a non-specific symptom and may be the presenting manifestation of a large number of disorders (Table 17). However, the relatively short duration of symptoms in a previously fit young person makes some diagnoses (e.g. thyrotoxicosis, diabetes mellitus (DM)) more likely than others.

History of the presenting problem

Allow the patient to explain what her major concerns are, then adopt a systematic approach with direct questions to screen for potential diagnoses for which relevant information has not been forthcoming. The following are important:

Table 17 Causes of weight loss.

Type of disorder	Example
Hypermetabolic states	Thyrotoxicosis DM Acute sepsis/trauma
Anorexia of chronic disorders	Infections, e.g. gastrointestinal, HIV Systemic inflammatory disorders Malignancy, including lymphoma Addison's disease
Reduced calorie intake	Anorexia nervosa Upper gastrointestinal tract pathology, e.g. oesophageal stricture Neurological disorders, e.g. motor neurone disease
Malabsorption	Coeliac disease
Increased physical activity	Female athletic triad

DM, diabetes mellitus; HIV, human immunodeficiency virus.

• general symptoms—ask about other non-specific symptoms such as fever, night sweats, lymphadenopathy. Lymphoma is not uncommon in this age group and weight loss constitutes one of the classical B symptoms
• appetite and calorie intake—what is her attitude to eating and to her loss of weight? Appetite may be increased in hypermetabolic states, reduced in true anorexia of chronic disorders, and is usually normal in anorexia nervosa where the problem is food refusal. Has she ever made herself vomit?
• abdominal symptoms—ask about dysphagia, vomiting/ regurgitation, abdominal pain or distension, and regarding bowel habit (frequency, consistency, blood, mucus, difficulty flushing).

It may be that a clear lead will emerge to suggest malignancy, malabsorption or anorexia nervosa: these possibilities should be pursued as indicated in *Gastroenterology and hepatology*, Section 1.10 and *Psychiatry*, Section 1.5. Is it possible that other conditions listed in Table 17 are present? In this young woman consider the following.

Thyrotoxicosis

Ask specifically about:
• heat intolerance. Does the patient need fewer/thinner clothes/bedclothes than those around her?
• goitre. Has there been any swelling or tenderness in the neck? Check for difficulty with swallowing/breathing
• palpitations, breathlessness
• tiredness, weakness, difficulty with sleeping
• menses, especially oligomenorrhoea/amenorrhoea
• mood—this woman has been getting into arguments: patients with thyrotoxicosis often report feeling unusually anxious/irritable/bad tempered

• bowel habit, particularly increased frequency
• recent pregnancy (consider postpartum thyroiditis)
• family history of autoimmune disease
• eye symptoms, e.g. prominence, dryness/itching, double vision.

Diabetes mellitus

Elicit further symptoms, e.g. polyuria, polydipsia, tiredness and lethargy.

Relevant past history

Is there is any history of previous surgery (especially abdominal) or chronic illness? Enquire about recent travel abroad. If you suspect anorexia nervosa, concentrate on taking a careful social history. Ask about alcohol consumption and smoking—the latter can exacerbate dysthyroid eye disease.

Autoimmune thyroid disease may be associated with other organ-specific autoimmune conditions, hence enquire about a personal or family history of thyroid disorders, DM, Addison's disease, pernicious anaemia, premature ovarian failure (POF) and vitiligo (see Section 2.7, p. 115).

Examination

The diagnosis may be apparent from general inspection:
• an anxious-looking, restless woman with warm sweaty hands, staring gaze and tremor has thyrotoxicosis until proved otherwise
• buccal and palmar pigmentation are suggestive of Addison's disease.

Check carefully for lymphadenopathy and clubbing and perform a thorough examination of the major systems to look for evidence of any malignancy, chronic cardiovascular or respiratory illnesses, gastrointestinal disorders, e.g. inflammatory bowel disease or malabsorption syndromes, chronic liver disease, alcoholism and neurological disorders including demyelinating disease. In particular: 'has this woman got thyrotoxicosis'?

 Physical signs in thyrotoxicosis

• Hands—fine tremor, warmth, acropachy (similar to clubbing)
• Pulse—tachycardia, atrial fibrillation
• Eyes—lid retraction and lid lag, proptosis, ophthalmopegia, periorbital oedema, chemosis (Fig. 12 and Section 2.3.2, p. 70)
• Neck—see Section 1.19, p. 43 for details regarding examination of the thyroid gland
• Skin—pretibial myxoedema
• Musculoskeletal—proximal myopathy.

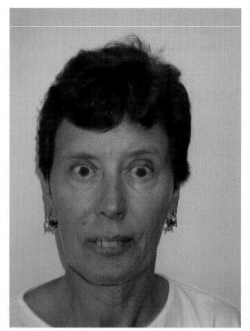

Fig. 12 Graves' disease. Note the typical 'staring eyes' with evidence of lid retraction and mild periorbital oedema.

Physical signs in DM

There may be little to find in a newly diagnosed type 1 diabetic aside from evidence of weight loss or secondary infection, e.g. candida.

Approach to investigation and management

Investigations

This should begin with 'screening tests' that are indicated in all cases of weight loss where the cause is not obvious.

Screening tests

Full blood count and CRP/erythrocyte sedimentation rate (ESR) (anaemia, infection, inflammation), urea and electrolytes (Addison's disease, anorexia nervosa, chronic renal impairment), fasting glucose, liver chemistry and calcium (intrinsic liver disease, malignancy), haematinics (ferritin, folate, vitamin B_{12}), and TSH. Check chest radiograph (lymphadenopathy, malignancy).

Further investigations should be directed by the findings on history, examination and screening tests. If these suggest:
- gastrointestinal disease: see *Gastroenterology and hepatology*, Section 1.10
- an eating disorder: see *Psychiatry*, Section 1.5.

Thyroid function tests

If you suspect thyroid disease, check:
- Free thyroxine (FT_4) ± free triiodothyronine (FT_3)
- TSH
- thyroid autoantibody titres (see Section 2.3.2, p. 70).

Radioisotope scans are not routinely performed in most centres, but may help to differentiate between the various aetiologies of hyperthyroidism when the clinical picture is not clear (e.g. in the absence of dysthyroid eye disease) (see Section 2.3.2, p. 70). The presence of a retrosternal goitre and associated tracheal compression/deviation may be evident on plain radiography (Fig. 13a) and can be confirmed if necessary by ultrasound (Fig. 13b) and/or flow volume loop analysis.

Other specific investigations

- Addison's disease—see Section 2.2.2, p. 59.
- lymphoma—see *Haematology*, Section 2.2
- human immunodeficiency virus (HIV)—this diagnosis will need to be considered if no other explanation for weight loss emerges. The question will need to be approached carefully: see *General clinical issues*, Section 2; *Infectious diseases*, Section 1.24.

Management

Thyrotoxicosis

The various available treatment options are discussed in detail in Section 2.3.2 (p. 72). Reassure the patient that she has a treatable condition that is not malignant. It is important to point out, however, that she might not feel 'completely back to normal' for some time, whilst fine adjustments are made to the medication. It may be useful to explain the concept of an autoimmune disease. For a woman of child-bearing age, as in this case, it is important to find out whether she could be pregnant or is planning a pregnancy in the near future, as this limits your treatment options (see Section 2.3.2, p. 74).

Other specific disorders

- DM—Section 2.6, p. 100.
- Addison's disease—Section 2.2.2, p. 59.
- Anorexia nervosa—see *Psychiatry*, Section 1.5
- Malabsorption—see *Gastroenterology and hepatology*, Section 2.6
- Inflammatory bowel disease—see *Gastroenterology and hepatology*, Section 2.1
- Lymphoma—see *Haematology*, Section 2.2
- HIV—see *Infectious diseases*, Section 2.11.

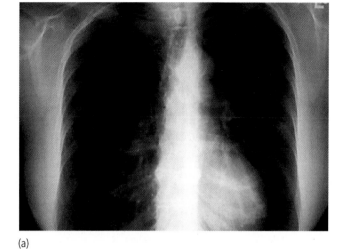

(a)

Fig. 13 Retrosternal goitre with tracheal compression. Chest radiograph (a) and thyroid ultrasound (b) showing tracheal narrowing by a large retrosternal goitre. Normal tracheal dimensions for comparison (c)!

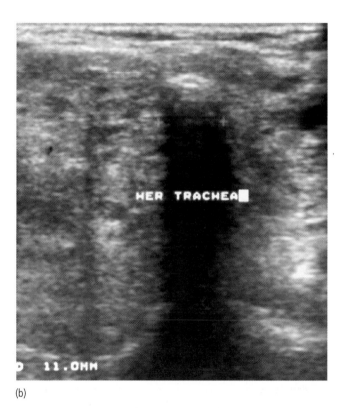

(b)

(c)

1.14 Tiredness and lethargy

Case history

A 54-year-old businessman is no longer able to meet the demands of his job, complaining of excessive tiredness, lethargy and altered bowel habit. The only past medical history of note is that of palpitations, which are now well controlled on amiodarone.

Clinical approach

Tiredness and lethargy are non-specific symptoms which

most of us experience from time to time—just think of the average junior doctor! The differential diagnosis is broad, including those conditions listed in Table 18.

History of the presenting problem

Tiredness and lethargy

Exactly what does the patient mean by 'tiredness and lethargy'? When did the symptoms first appear? Have they been continuous or intermittent? Do they stop them doing anything that they would like to do? What activities have they had to cut out? If the problem is that they fall asleep every night at 7.00 pm, then this is certainly unusual; if it means that they are unable to sustain working from 7.00 am until

Table 18 Disorders presenting with tiredness and lethargy.

Type of condition	Common or important example
'Normal variant'	Hard work
	Childcare
Psychological/psychiatric disorder	Anxiety
	Depression
	Alcohol dependence
	Chronic fatigue syndrome
Chronic/systemic illness, usually obvious in this context	Malignancy
	Heart failure
	Respiratory failure
Systemic illness, not always obvious	Anaemia
	Thyroid deficiency (or occasionally excess)
	Diabetes mellitus
	Primary hyperparathyroidism
	Addison's disease

midnight for 5 or 6 nights a week for very long, then few are able to do this and they expect too much of themselves.

Change of bowel habit

The matter of change in bowel habit clearly needs to be explored, and the history should encompass a full systems enquiry to check for leads to any of the conditions listed in Table 18. Talk about 'physical' symptoms and problems before moving on to 'psychological/pyschiatric' issues. The following possibilities should be considered as the history is taken.

Anaemia

Is there any history of indigestion or peptic ulcer disease? Elicit further details regarding the altered bowel habit (see *Gastroenterology and hepatology*, Section 1.11). Consider other causes of anaemia (see *Haematology*, Sections 1.1, 1.3 and 1.4).

Thyroid disease

Both hypo- and hyperthyroidism (Section 2.3.1, p. 67) can present in this manner. This is likely to be of particular importance in this case since the patient is on amiodarone, which can be associated with hypo- or hyperthyroidism (Fig. 14). Although unlikely, consider the possibility that his original palpitations were a manifestation of thyroid hormone excess, now followed by thyroid hormone deficiency (a feature of thyroiditis—Section 2.3.2, p. 72).

Diabetes mellitus

Excessive tiredness and lethargy are well recognized presenting features of diabetes. Elicit further symptoms including polyuria, polydipsia and weight loss.

The anti-arrhythmic agent amiodarone has a high organic iodine content (approximately $1/3$ by weight) and bears structural similarities to both T_4 and T_3:

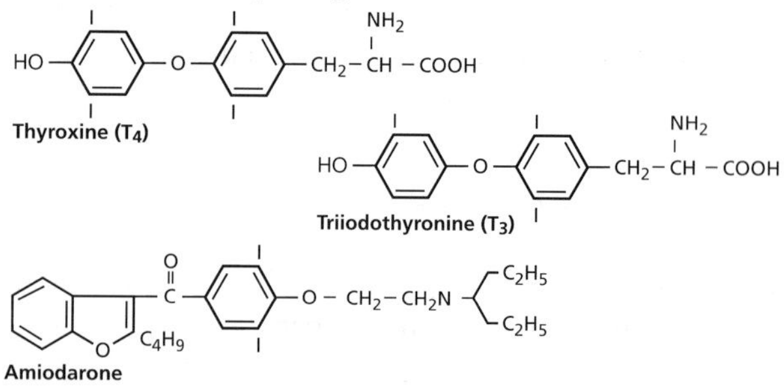

Standard maintenance doses of amiodarone (100–200 mg/day) result in a massive expansion of the iodide pool and can influence thyroid physiology in various ways:

1 Abnormalities of thyroid function in clinically euthyroid individuals:
- $\uparrow T_4$ and rT_3 ⎤
- $\downarrow T_3$ ⎦ through inhibition of the type 1 deiodinase
- $\uparrow$ TSH during early stages of treatment (? an effect on the pituitary type 2 deiodinase)

In the absence of overt symptoms of thyroid disease, specific treatment is usually not required, but thyroid function tests should be monitored periodically.

2 Amiodarone-induced thyrotoxicosis occurs in some patients and can arise through several mechanisms including:
- stimulation of excess hormone synthesis in response to an iodine load (more common in iodine deficient regions and may represent unmasking of occult thyroid disease, the so-called Jod–Basedow effect)
- destruction of thyroid follicles with subsequent release of thyroid hormones (essentially an inflammatory thyroiditis). Treatment can be difficult since it is often not possible to stop amiodarone. Medical therapy including antithyroid drugs and glucocorticoids may be necessary, with surgery reserved for difficult cases.

3 Amiodarone-induced hypothyroidism is more common in iodine-replete areas and in those with detectable thyroid autoantibodies. Again various mechanisms have been invoked, including the Wolff–Chaikoff effect in which high intra-thyroidal iodide concentrations inhibit thyroid hormone biosynthesis. Treatment is generally easier than for thyrotoxicosis since amiodarone can be continued if necessary, and T_4 replacement therapy given.

Accordingly, it is wise to check thyroid function tests (FT_4, FT_3 and TSH) prior to commencing amiodarone and to periodically repeat them during treatment. Moreover, in light of its long half-life, abnormalities of thyroid function may persist for several months after discontinuation of therapy.

Fig. 14 Amiodarone and thyroid function.

Adrenal insufficiency

Tiredness and lethargy may be the only presenting symptoms of hypoadrenalism (Section 2.2.2, p. 59).

Primary hyperparathyroidism

Tiredness and constipation are common manifestations of chronic hypercalcaemia. Has the patient had urinary stones?

Anxiety and depression

Ask about the physical manifestations of depressive illness such as early morning wakening and poor appetite; also regarding the psychological/social factors that may be causative, e.g. stress at the office/home.

Chronic fatigue syndrome

This is a difficult diagnosis that remains one of exclusion. Ask about poor concentration and memory, irritability, altered sleep and muscle aches.

Relevant past history

This should include details of chronic/systemic illness; any autoimmune illnesses in the patient or their family; other medication, for example β-blockers; alcohol consumption.

Examination

Your overall impression of the patient is important:
- Does he seem anxious or depressed?
- Is he anaemic?
- Are there features of chronic/systemic upset, e.g. wasting/cachexia?
- Is there any lymphadenopathy?

A full physical examination is required. Given that the only symptom that points to an organ system is change in bowel habit, check specifically for abdominal masses or hepatomegaly and perform a rectal examination ± proctoscopy/sigmoidoscopy.

Specifically consider those conditions listed in Table 18:
- thyroid disease—assess thyroid status, looking for evidence of a goitre and for signs of hypo- or hyperthyroidism (see Sections 1.13, p. 29 and 2.3.1, p. 67)
- DM—examine specifically for evidence of complications, which are often present at the time of diagnosis of type 2 diabetes (see Section 2.6, p. 100)
- hypoadrenalism—is the patient pigmented? Check for a postural fall in BP (see Section 2.2.2, p. 59)
- primary hyperparathyroidism—hypercalcaemia rarely produces signs, but band keratopathy may be evident (see Section 2.5.7, p. 95).

Physical signs in hypothyroidism

- Lethargy
- Husky voice
- Puffy face and hands
- Cold dry skin
- Goitre
- Slow-relaxing reflexes.

Approach to investigation and management

Investigations

Some simple screening tests are required, even in the absence of specific symptoms and signs.

Screening tests

Check full blood count (anaemia), electrolytes and renal function (chronic renal impairment, Addison's disease), liver chemistry and calcium (chronic liver disease, metastases, hypercalcaemia), fasting glucose and thyroid function tests (TFTs). Check chest radiograph (malignancy).

Further tests

Further investigations should be directed by the findings on history, examination and screening tests:
- gastrointestinal disease—see *Gastroenterology and hepatology*, Sections 1.10 and 1.15.
- anaemia—see *Haematology*, Section 2.1
- hypo- and hyperthyroidism (see Section 2.3), DM (see Section 2.6), hypoadrenalism (see Section 2.2.2, p. 59), primary hyperparathyroidism (see Section 2.5.7, p. 95).

Management

- Gastrointestinal disease—see *Gastroenterology and hepatology*, Sections 1.10 and 1.15
- Anaemia—the underlying aetiology determines appropriate specific treatment (see *Haematology*, Section 2.1)
- Hypo- and hyperthyroidism (see Section 2.3), DM (see Section 2.6), hypoadrenalism (see Section 2.2.2, p. 59), primary hyperparathyroidism (see Section 2.5.7, p. 95). An approach to the management of amiodarone-induced thyroid dysfunction, the diagnosis in this case, is shown in Fig. 14
- Anxiety/depression/alcohol dependence—see *Psychiatry*, Sections 2.7 and 2.11.

 Loh KC. Amiodarone-induced thyroid disorders: a clinical review. *Postgrad Med J* 2000; 76(893): 133–140.

1.15 Flushing and diarrhoea

Case history

A 50-year-old man is referred to Out-patients early in the New Year. He has been unable to enjoy the festive season at all, as any over-indulgence has resulted in severe facial flushing. He has also been troubled by rather watery diarrhoea.

Clinical approach

Although it is important to bear in mind the possibility that the symptoms are unrelated, taken together they suggest a number of specific diagnoses.

Conditions associated with 'flushing and diarrhoea'

- Anxiety attacks
- Diabetic autonomic neuropathy (gustatory sweating and diarrhoea)
- Thyrotoxicosis
- Carcinoid syndrome
- Phaeochromocytoma
- Systemic mastocytosis (rare).

History of the presenting problem

Flushing

Ask the patient to describe a typical flushing episode. Note in particular:
- frequency and duration of each attack
- distribution of flushing, e.g. face, trunk
- other precipitating factors, e.g. exercise
- associated symptoms, e.g. palpitations, sweating
- relevant drug history, e.g. calcium channel antagonists and the sulphonylurea chlorpropamide are recognized causes of facial flushing.

Diarrhoea

First find out what the patient considers to be his normal bowel habit, then:
- What does he mean by 'diarrhoea' (e.g. increased frequency of stool or loose motions)?
- Has there been any blood or mucus with the stool?
- What about precipitating factors, e.g. specific foods?
- What about recent travel abroad?
- Check for other systemic symptoms, e.g. weight loss.

Other symptoms

Bearing in mind the possible diagnoses listed above, ask about the following if the information is not forthcoming spontaneously.
- Anxiety attacks—these would almost certainly be the commonest cause of this presentation. Are there other features to support this diagnosis? Has has he had pins and needles affecting the hands and feet; 'atypical' chest pain; a history of medically unexplained symptoms?
- DM—gustatory sweating and altered bowel habit are recognized features of diabetic autonomic neuropathy, but this is a feature of long-established diabetes and not a presentation of this conditon (see Section 2.6, p. 100).
- Thyrotoxicosis—enquire about weight loss, heat intolerance, tremor, proximal myopathy, etc. (see Section 2.3.2, p. 70).

- Carcinoid syndrome—the majority of carcinoid tumours arise from enterochromaffin cells of the intestine. In general, they are slow growing and many are asymptomatic until metastases develop. Carcinoid syndrome only occurs when there are hepatic metastases or (rarely) a pulmonary primary releasing 5-hydroxytryptamine (5-HT) directly into the systemic circulation (thereby circumventing first pass metabolism in the liver). It commonly leads to flushing (which may be spontaneous or precipitated by food, alcohol or stress) and recurrent watery diarrhoea. Other less common characteristics include abdominal pain, wheeze, right-sided heart disease and pellagra (dermatitis, diarrhoea and dementia due to niacin deficiency).
- Phaeochromocytoma—ask about related symptoms, e.g. anxiety, palpitations, hypertension.

Examination

First impressions count! However, do not be tempted to ascribe the symptoms to simple anxiety until you have excluded other causes. This man is entitled to be anxious about his condition: furthermore, anxiety is a manifestation of several of the differential diagnoses under consideration. Does he look as though he has lost weight? Is he pale? Is there lymphadenopathy?

Gastrointestinal

Check carefully for masses and organomegaly. A rectal examination including proctoscopy and sigmoidoscopy is essential in view of the altered bowel habit.

Other systems

As with the history, consider the differential diagnosis as you examine the patient:
- DM—in a diabetic with this presentation, look carefully for other complications of diabetes including retinopathy, microalbuminuria/proteinuria, peripheral neuropathy, hypertension, vascular bruits/absent pulses. Check for postural hypotension and loss of sinus dysrhythmia—both features of autonomic neuropathy
- thyrotoxicosis—check if there a goitre, dysthyroid eye disease, resting tachycardia, tremor, etc. (see Sections 1.13, p. 28 and 2.3.2, p. 70)
- carcinoid syndrome—find the jugular venous pulse, feel for a right ventricular heave, listen in the pulmonary area and left parasternal region for pulmonary valve murmurs. Right heart valvular lesions, e.g. pulmonary stenosis, are a recognized complication: you'll never spot them if you don't examine with this in mind
- phaeochromocytoma—check for hypertension and postural hypotension.

Approach to investigation and management

Investigations

Screening tests required include full blood count, electrolytes, renal and liver function, fasting glucose, thyroid function, inflammatory markers (ESR and/or CRP), and a chest radiograph.

Other investigations should be guided by the patient's presentation:
- DM (see Section 2.6, p. 100)
- thyrotoxicosis (see Section 2.3.2, p. 70)
- phaeochromocytoma (see Section 2.2.5, p. 65).

In this patient there were no firm leads to these conditions after history, examination and sceening investigations, and attention focused on the possibility of carcinoid syndrome.

Carcinoid syndrome

To look for biochemical and structural evidence the following investigations are appropriate:
- 24-h urinary 5-hydroxyindoleacetic acid (5-HIAA) excretion—5-HIAA is a metabolite of 5-HT. A 24-h collection is a sensitive (~75%) and specific (approaching 100%) test for carcinoid syndrome
- ultrasound/CT—once the diagnosis has been confirmed biochemically, the liver should be imaged with ultrasound or CT. If the liver is clear, perform a chest CT to look for a pulmonary primary
- octreoscan—using radiolabelled octreotide approximately 85% of tumours can be visualized (Fig. 15). Uptake indicates that the tumour may respond to treatment with somatostatin analogues.

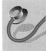
The carcinoid primary

Note that unless a primary carcinoid tumour is causing symptoms in its own right (e.g. intestinal obstruction), there is usually little to be gained in undertaking a protracted search to localize it.

Management

This will clearly be dependant on the particular diagnosis:
- anxiety/panic attacks—the patient may respond to reassurance that there is no sinister diagnosis, but consider referral for specialist psychological/psychiatric input if symptoms are persistent and intrusive (see *Psychiatry*, Sections 1.6 and 2.7)
- DM—see Section 2.6, p. 100
- thyrotoxicosis—see Section 2.3.2, p. 70
- phaeochromocytoma—see Section 2.2.5, p. 65.

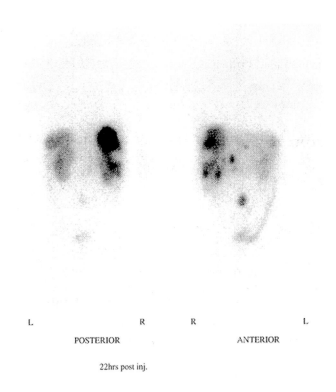

L   R   R   L

POSTERIOR   ANTERIOR

22hrs post inj.

Fig. 15 Octreoscan. Radiolabelled octreotide scan demonstrating focal uptake centrally within the abdomen (primary tumour) and multiple areas of hepatic uptake (metastases) in a 67-year-old man with carcinoid syndrome.

Carcinoid syndrome

COMMUNICATION

This man should be given the opportunity of patient and careful explanation of his condition. Carcinoid tumours can fall anywhere along a spectrum from indolent to highly malignant: this degree of uncertainty is difficult for both patients and doctors to deal with (see *General clinical issues*, Section 2). Survival for 10–15 years is not uncommon, but it is uncertain whether any of the treatment options outlined below affect life expectancy. The condition is rare, few doctors have much experience of it, and it is best managed in a specialist centre. This, however, may have obvious inconveniences—e.g. lengthy travel, admission to hospital far from home—and these issues will need to be thought through and discussed.

LIFESTYLE AND SIMPLE REMEDIES

Patients may be able to identify precipitating factors that they can avoid, such as alcohol, spicy food or strenuous exercise. Symptomatic treatment of diarrhoea with loperamide is worthwhile. Nicotinic acid supplements (i.e. multivitamin tablets) should be recommended. Antihistamines with antiserotoninergic activity (e.g. cyproheptadine) may be useful. Asthma (if present) can be treated with inhaled β-agonists.

SURGERY

Symptomatic primaries and occasionally single hepatic metastases (depending on their size and position) may be amenable to resection.

SOMATOSTATIN ANALOGUES

Octreotide and the longer acting somatostatin analogues frequently relieve symptoms of flushing and diarrhoea, although there is little evidence that they inhibit tumour growth. Unfortunately they have to be given by injection, and side-effects may include diarrhoea, nausea/vomiting and gallstones. Intravenous octreotide is useful in the event of a carcinoid crisis (see below).

CHEMOTHERAPY

Chemotherapy (e.g. 5-fluorouracil; interferon-α) has a limited role in the treatment of patients with carcinoid syndrome as the benefits are often outweighed by the side-effects.

SELECTIVE EMBOLIZATION VIA THE HEPATIC ARTERY

The premise for hepatic artery embolization is that tumours receive most of their blood supply from the hepatic artery, whilst hepatocytes are also able to derive blood from the portal venous circulation. Selective embolization should be undertaken in specialist centres only. The patient is likely to experience fever, pain and nausea. Treatment may precipitate a carcinoid crisis (hypotension, tachycardia and bronchoconstriction), and carries with it a risk of massive hepatic necrosis.

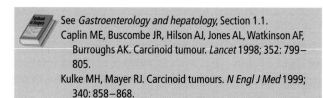

See *Gastroenterology and hepatology*, Section 1.1.
Caplin ME, Buscombe JR, Hilson AJ, Jones AL, Watkinson AF, Burroughs AK. Carcinoid tumour. *Lancet* 1998; 352: 799–805.
Kulke MH, Mayer RJ. Carcinoid tumours. *N Engl J Med* 1999; 340: 858–868.

1.16 'Off legs'

Case history

A 72-year-old woman is admitted as an emergency 'off legs'. Until recently she has been independent, able to do her own shopping and refusing home help. Over the last few months, however, she has developed widespread aches and pains and increasing immobility, with particular difficulty getting to her feet. Her past medical history is unremarkable

Table 19 Conditions associated with a proximal myopathy.

Type of disorder	Example
Muscle disease	Polymyositis/dermatomyositis Infective myositis Inherited muscular dystrophies
Metabolic and endocrine disease	Diabetic amyotrophy Osteomalacia Cushing's syndrome Thyrotoxicosis (and occasionally hypothyroidism) Glycogen and lipid storage diseases
Malignancy	Carcinomatous neuropathy
Drug induced	Alcohol Glucocorticoids

apart from long-standing idiopathic epilepsy that is well controlled on treatment. She is not febrile or confused.

Clinical approach

The differential diagnosis of immobility in the elderly is broad. The principal clue in this history is the suggestion of a proximal myopathy. The history, examination and investigation should be directed at confirming this, whilst excluding other causes of weakness, and establishing the underlying diagnosis (Table 19). Polymyalgia rheumatica is a common cause of aches and pains in the elderly, predominantly involving the muscles of the shoulder and pelvic girdle, and clearly needs to be considered. A particular clue to the diagnosis in this case could be the history of epilepsy and long-term anticonvulsant therapy, raising the possibility of osteomalacia.

History of the presenting problem

Given the wide range of causes of weakness in the elderly, and of proximal myopathy in particular, a full history is needed, beginning with careful consideration of the symptoms themselves:

Weakness, aches and pains

The brief details given suggest that weakness might be due to proximal myopathy: the first priority is to confirm that weakness is indeed present, and that limitation of movement is not simply caused by pain. It would be misleading to probe extensively for causes of proximal myopathy if, in fact, the problem was due to lumbar back pain with nerve root irritation. Ask carefully about the following if the details do not emerge spontaneously.
• Is the problem in one or both legs? If the problem is much worse in one leg than the other, then a myopathic condition is unlikely and attention should focus on 'local'

disorders, e.g. spinal pain with nerve root irritation; undeclared hip fracture

• How did the problem start? Onset after a fall would suggest a traumatic cause of pain, perhaps fracture of a lumbar vertebra or hip

• Which things are most difficult to do? When is the weakness most noticeable? With proximal myopathy there is particular difficulty when rising from a chair or on climbing stairs. With rheumatic disorders, e.g. rheumatoid arthritis, there may be diurnal variation, with pain and stiffness worst in the morning and then improving as the patient 'warms up'

• What is the distribution of aches and pains? Pain in the affected muscles is suggestive of an inflammatory myositis or diabetic amyotrophy. Pain in a radicular distribution suggests nerve root irritation (see *Neurology*, Section 1.2). Generalized aches and pains are in keeping with osteomalacia, and also with the much commoner condition of polymyalgia rheumatica. Polymyalgia rheumatica does not, however, cause weakness, although pain and stiffness in the affected muscle groups may be perceived as such. Are there any other symptoms to support this diagnosis? Ask about headaches, scalp tenderness, visual symptoms and jaw claudication (see *Medicine for the elderly*, Section 1.5; *Ophthalmology*, Section 1.5; *Rheumatology and clinical immunology*, Section 2.5.1).

Neurological symptoms

Weakness could clearly have a primarily neurological cause. Focal symptoms, e.g. weakness of one leg rather than both in this case, would clearly imply focal pathology, e.g. unrecognized stroke. The presence of sensory, e.g. numbness and paraesthesia, would suggest neuropathy rather than myopathy (see *Neurology*, Section 1.1).

Other symptoms

A full systems enquiry is needed, bearing particularly in mind the diagnoses listed in Table 19 given that enquiries along the lines indicated above regarding the pain and weakness did suggest that a myopathic problem was likely in this case.

• Polymyositis/dermatomyositis—ask about arthralgia/arthritis, especially affecting the small joints of the hand (~50% of cases), and rashes, e.g. the heliotrope rash of dermatomyositis (see *Rheumatology and clinical immunology*, Sections 1.15 and 2.3.5)

• Diabetic amyotrophy—typically seen in older patients (especially men), who present with asymmetrical weakness and wasting of the quadriceps muscles. Ask about pain in the thigh, which often keeps the patient awake at night

• Osteomalacia—a history of long-term anticonvulsant use (phenytoin or barbiturates, as in this case) but also of renal disease, previous gastric surgery, coeliac disease or other malabsorptive states should prompt consideration

of osteomalacia. The elderly and Asian populations are at particular risk, reflecting reduced skin synthesis of vitamin D together with dietary insufficiency (see Section 2.5.5, p. 92)

• Cushing's syndrome—many of the features of Cushing's syndrome (e.g. easy bruising, thin skin, weight gain) may be mistaken for part of the 'normal ageing process'

• Thyroid disease—ask about the classical symptoms of thyrotoxicosis and hypothyroidism (see Section 2.3.1, p. 67), but remember that the clinical features may be modified in the elderly.

Relevant past medical history

Check for a history of asthma, arthritis or other illnesses requiring long-term corticosteroid treatment. Ask about alcohol intake: this could be a 'pseudo-Cushing's' presentation (see Section 2.1.1, p. 47).

Examination

> **Examination of weakness and pain**
>
> *Is there weakness, or is limitation due to the fact that movement is painful?*
> Most patients who are admitted 'off legs' have had an acute event such as a stroke or an acute infective illness, e.g. urinary tract infection. Given the wide differential diagnosis of this presentation, a full physical examination is required, beginning with the vital signs and looking for evidence of infection. There was no suggestion from the history that this was this woman's problem and attention focused directly on causes of musculoskeletal pain and weakness.

Musculoskeletal and neurological

• Could this be an acute presentation of a rheumatic disorder? Is there arthritis or local bone tenderness (see *Rheumatology and clinical immunology*, Sections 1.19, 1.22 and 1.23)? Are the temporal arteries tender (see *Rheumatology and clinical immunology*, Section 2.5.1)? Tenderness of the muscles suggests myositis

• Is there weakness, and what is its distribution? Weakness tends to be more marked proximally in myopathy and distally in neuropathy. In proximal myopathy, observing the patient stand from a chair or squatting position can be very informative

• Look for signs suggestive of a neuropathic, nerve root, spinal cord or pyramidal pattern of disease (see *Neurology*, Section 1.2).

Myopathy

This woman appeared to have a myopathy, hence it was appropriate to look specifically for evidence pointing to any of the conditions listed in Table 19:

• heliotrope rash (dermatomyositis; see *Rheumatology and clinical immunology*, Section 2.3.5)
• thyroid disease (see Section 2.3, p. 67)
• DM (see Section 2.6, p. 100)
• Cushing's syndrome (see Section 2.1.1, p. 47).

Approach to investigation and management

Investigations

Having established the presence of a proximal myopathy, the principal aim of investigation is to establish the cause.

General

Many of the causes of proximal myopathy can be screened for with routine blood tests including:
• Full blood count—anaemia suggestive of chronic disease or iron deficiency
• ESR/CRP—raised in inflammatory muscle diseases
• Urea and electrolytes—renal failure; familial periodic paralysis
• Fasting glucose
• Creatine kinase—raised in inflammatory muscle disease and hypothyroidism
• Liver chemistry—low albumin in malabsorption, raised alkaline phosphatase in osteomalacia
• Ca^{2+}, PO_4^{2-}—low/low normal in osteomalacia
• TSH—suppressed in thyrotoxicosis and elevated in hypothyroidism.

Further investigations

Other tests that may be indicated include:
• PTH—raised in osteomalacia, renal osteodystrophy
• vitamin D–25(OH)D_3 is typically low in osteomalacia, although 1,25(OH)$_2D_3$ may be normal
• when malabsorption is suspected: serum ferritin to look for iron deficiency, prothrombin time to screen for vitamin K malabsorption, antigliadin and antiendomysial antibodies as indicators of coeliac disease
• 24-h urinary free cortisol estimation or dexamethasone suppression if there is evidence of Cushing's syndrome
• radiological studies if osteomalacia is suspected (see Section 2.5.5, p. 92).

If these investigations fail to identify a cause for the proximal myopathy, consider further tests including electromyography and/or muscle biopsy.

Management

If, as in this case, investigation confirms osteomalacia, treatment is with vitamin D supplementation (see Section 2.5.5, p. 93). In cases of renal failure or malabsorption the vitamin D metabolites alfacalcidol or calcitriol are usually required, often with dietary calcium supplements. Other causes of proximal myopathy should be treated according to the underlying diagnosis:
• polymyositis/dermatomyositis (see *Rheumatology and clinical immunology*, Sections 1.15 and 2.3.5)
• thyroid disease (see Section 2.3, p. 67)
• DM (see Section 2.6, p. 100)
• Cushing's syndrome (see Section 2.1.1, p. 47).

 See *Medicine for the elderly*, Sections 1.1 and 1.5. Francis RM, Selby PL. Osteomalacia. *Baillière's Clin Endocrinol Metab* 1997; 11: 145–163.

1.17 Avoiding another coronary

Case history

A 52-year-old male company director is reviewed in clinic following a recent myocardial infarction. He is currently being treated with aspirin and atenolol and has completed a normal exercise test. His cholesterol is 4.2 and he is keen to know what more can be done to prevent a further heart attack.

Clinical approach

The aim must be to identify all modifiable risk factors and address them in discussion with the patient.

History of the presenting problem

In taking the history you will obviously discuss symptoms of vascular disease and enquire about further episodes of chest pain, evidence of cardiac failure (has he had shortness of breath, orthopnoea or swelling of his ankles?) and any symptoms of cerebrovascular or peripheral vascular disease. These enquiries do not produce any positive replies, and attention moves to risk factors.
• Diet—is he on any sort of diet? What did he have to eat yesterday? Was this a typical day? Note consumption of saturated fat and also ask specifically about dietary/vitamin supplements, e.g. antioxidant vitamins, folic acid, ω-3 unsaturated fatty acids (fish oil), and alcohol consumption.
• Exercise—does he take regular exercise? If yes, how much and how often?
• Smoking—is he still smoking?
• Other risk factors—check for a history of diabetes and/or hypertension. Do heart attacks or other vascular problems run in the family?

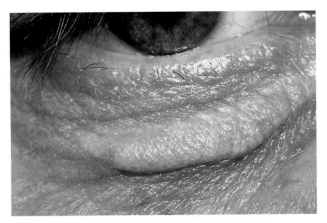

Fig. 16 Xanthelasma.

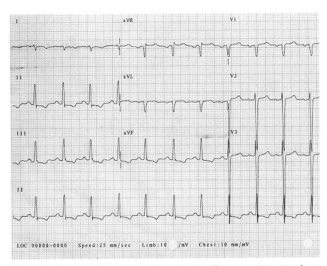

Fig. 17 Left ventricular hypertrophy. Note the tall R waves in V_5–V_6, deep S in V_2 and inverted T waves in II, III, aVF, V_5–V_6.

In this particular case, the man's diet was reasonable with an alcohol consumption of approximately 21 U per week. He had taken little exercise since his youth, and had been told that his BP was 'borderline' for several years. He had successfully stopped smoking 10 years before his heart attack. There was no family history of note.

Examination

In all patients with ischaemic heart disease (IHD) a full examination should be performed, paying particular attention to:
• stigmata of hyperlipidaemia and hypertension (Fig. 16) (see Section 1.18, p. 40)
• weight and height to allow calculation of BMI
• cardiovascular and respiratory systems—pulse, BP, bruits, murmurs, signs of cardiac failure, peripheral pulses
• evidence of liver or kidney disease, DM, thyroid disease.
In this case, his BMI was 32 kg/m², BP 160/95, and silver wiring was noted on fundoscopy.

Approach to investigation and management

Investigations

Baseline 'screening' blood tests should include full blood count, electrolytes, renal and liver function, fasting glucose and fasting full lipid profile.

If not already performed, it would be appropriate to check an ECG and chest radiograph (and perhaps an echocardiogram) to provide a baseline assessment of the heart, looking in particular for evidence of left ventricular hypertrophy (Fig. 17) or dysfunction.

In this case, the fasting glucose was 6.5 and a subsequent OGTT (see Section 3.1.7, p. 121) showed evidence of impaired glucose tolerance. The total cholesterol was 4.2, with high density lipoprotein (HDL) cholesterol of 0.7, giving a ratio of 6.0. The low density lipoproteins (LDL) cholesterol was 3.0 and triglycerides were 2.5.

Metabolic syndrome X

The combination of hypertension, impaired glucose tolerance (indicating insulin resistance), mixed dyslipidaemia and obesity constitutes the metabolic syndrome (also known as Reaven's syndrome or syndrome X), which is now recognized to be associated with a high risk of IHD.

Management

What can this man do to help himself, and what can be done for him?
• Diet—refer to a dietician to ensure that the diet is low in saturated fat (red meat, dairy products, egg yolks, fried food); low in refined carbohydrates; reduced in calories (to promote weight loss); and high in antioxidant vitamins, folic acid, ω-3 fatty acids (fresh fruit and green vegetables and oily fish)
• Exercise—advise moderate exercise (walking, swimming, cycling) for 30–40 min 3–4 times per week
• Weight reduction—usually best achieved through a combination of dietary modification and increased exercise
• BP control—target ≤140/80–85
• Lipid lowering—aiming to achieve LDL cholesterol <3 mmol/L; HDL cholesterol >1 mmol/L; triglycerides <2.0 mmol/L.

Whilst dietary change, increased exercise and weight reduction might achieve satisfactory control of BP and lipids in time, more aggressive treatment (e.g. with an ACE inhibitor and a statin or fibrate) is warranted in the presence of established IHD, as in this man. BP and lipid status should be monitored periodically, and relatives offered screening for cardiovascular risk factors. He is already on aspirin and a β-blocker for secondary prevention.

Treatment of metabolic syndrome X

When treating individual components of this condition, bear in mind the other aspects, e.g. try to avoid antihypertensive agents that have adverse effects on lipids or blood sugar (e.g. bendrofluazide).

Reaven GM. Role of insulin resistance in human disease (syndrome X): an expanded definition. *Annu Rev Med* 1993; 44: 121.

1.18 High blood pressure and low serum potassium

Case history

A 40-year-old man has been referred for advice. Hypertension (160/105) was diagnosed 6 months earlier when he presented with generalized weakness and tiredness. Blood tests have shown that he is not anaemic, but his serum potassium is 2.4 mmol/L, and the GP asks whether he might have Conn's syndrome in the referral letter.

Clinical approach

Although essential hypertension can strike at any age, a concern in any young patient presenting with high BP is to exclude a secondary cause (Table 20). The tiredness and weakness, although non-specific, are probably related to hypokalaemia in this case and would favour some of the secondary causes, including the primary hyperaldosteronism suggested by the GP.

Table 20 Causes of secondary hypertension.

Type of condition	Example
Renal	Parenchymal disease, e.g. glomerulonephritis, chronic pyelonephritis, polycystic kidney disease Renovascular disease, e.g. atheromatous renal artery stenosis
Endocrine	Primary hyperaldosteronism, e.g. Conn's syndrome Cushing's syndrome Primary hyperparathyroidism Acromegaly Phaeochromocytoma DM/insulin resistance (Reaven's syndrome)
Drugs	Corticosteroids, oral contraceptive pill
Others	Coarctation of aorta Pregnancy-associated hypertension

DM, diabetes mellitus.

History of the presenting problem

The history should obviously begin with brief discussion of the patient's symptoms of tiredness and weakness, also details of how his hypertension was discovered, and whether he had ever had his BP measured previously, before moving on to cover causes and consequences of both hypertension and hypokalaemia.

Causes of hypertension

Ask about the following if the details are not forthcoming:
- is there a family history of high BP? Does he know if his parents, brothers or sisters are on antihypertensive drugs? If they are, 'essential' hypertension becomes an even more likely diagnosis (although a rare familial form of hypertension would be an outside possibility)
- is there any history of renal disease? Has he had medicals for work or insurance where his urine has been checked in the past? A report of a 'just a bit of protein and/or blood' may indicate that he has long-standing renal disease and hypertension secondary to this
- could there be a phaeochromocytoma? This is the only one of the endocrine secondary causes where the diagnosis is likely to be made on the basis of the history. Most patients with phaeochromocytoma will have some symptoms suggestive of catecholamine excess, the commonest being headache, sweating, palpitations and episodes of pallor (see Section 2.2.5, p. 65).

It is most unlikely that the history will give clear clues to the other secondary causes of high BP listed in Table 20.

Consequences of hypertension

Have there been any symptoms related to target organ damage?
- Cardiac—chest pain/myocardial infarct, dyspnoea, peripheral oedema
- Cerebrovascular accidents/transient ischaemic attacks
- Retinopathy.

Causes of hypokalaemia

There are many causes of hypokalaemia (Table 21). Given that hypertension is common, it is possible that the hypokalaemia is not associated with it and therefore important to consider other explanations. Hence ask about the following:
- diarrhoea or vomiting
- diuretics (has he been prescribed these for his hypertension?)
- consumption of laxatives or liquorice
- proximal myopathy or other symptoms of steroid excess —hypokalaemia is most prominent in the setting of ectopic ACTH secretion. This is unlikely to be the diagnosis in this case with a 6-month history: the usual cause

Table 21 Causes of hypokalaemia.

Total body potassium	Mechanism	Common or important example
Normal	Shift of potassium into cells	β-Adrenergic stimulation Periodic paralysis
Reduced	Renal potassium wasting	Alkalosis, e.g. due to vomiting Diuretics Hyperaldosteronism Cushing's syndrome Liquorice addiction Genetic: Gitelman's, Bartter's syndromes Various renal tubular disorders
	Gastrointestinal potassium loss	Any cause of diarrhoea Intestinal fistulae Colonic villous adenoma

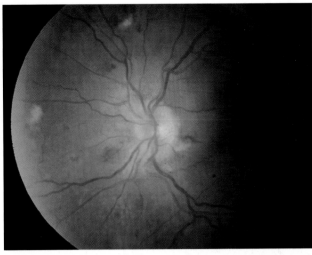

Fig. 18 Hypertensive retinopathy. Advanced retinal changes (cotton wool exudates, flame and blot haemorrhages, blurring of the optic disc margins) identified in a 50-year-old man with hypertensive cardiomyopathy.

is malignancy and the pace of deterioration rapid (see Section 2.1.1, p. 47)
• family history of 'a potassium problem'.

Remember that there are no clinical features beyond hypertension and symptoms related to hypokalaemia that might support the diagnosis of primary hyperaldosteronism: a high index of suspicion is needed to make the diagnosis.

Consequences of hypokalaemia

Enquire about other symptoms that might be due to hypokalaemia, e.g. thirst, polyuria (nephrogenic diabetes insipidus (DI)), paraesthesia (hypokalaemic alkalosis).

Relevant past history

In any patient with hypertension it is clearly important to enquire about other cardiovascular risk factors—smoking, cholesterol, DM and family history.

Examination

A thorough physical examination is required, paying particular attention to following aspects:
• pulse and BP? At least two readings 5 min apart; in addition, check lying and standing BP. Resting tachycardia, hypertension and postural hypotension may indicate phaeochromocytoma
• is there evidence of cardiac failure? Check jugular venous pressure; palpate apex (displaced); listen for mitral regurgitation (due to left ventricular dilatation) or gallop rhythm and basal crepitations; peripheral oedema
• is there evidence of left ventricular hypertrophy? Palpate apex (thrusting)
• is there coarctation? Feel for radio-femoral delay; listen for systolic murmur

• is there renovascular disease? Listen for bruits over carotid and femoral arteries and feel for abdominal aortic aneurysm and peripheral pulses (evidence of generalized atheromatous disease); listen for bruit over abdomen and in loins (may be due to renal artery stenosis)
• can you palpate the kidneys? They are not normally palpable, except in thin women, and if they can be felt consider adult polycystic kidney disease
• is there hypertensive retinopathy (Fig. 18)? See *Cardiology*, Section 2.17.

Approach to investigation and management

Investigations

Routine

HYPERTENSION

In any patient presenting with hypertension it would be appropriate to check the following:
• dipstick urinalysis, sending specimen for microscopy (casts) and culture if this shows proteinuria or haematuria
• full blood count—anaemia of chronic disease, e.g. renal failure
• electrolytes and renal function—to confirm hypokalaemia and look for renal failure
• random glucose, with subsequent fasting sample if abnormal—impaired glucose tolerance/DM is associated with acromegaly and Cushing's syndrome
• ECG/echocardiography—looking for changes of left ventricular hypertrophy seen with long-standing hypertension (Fig. 17, p. 39)
• chest radiograph—to look for evidence of cardiomegaly, pulmonary oedema or rib notching (coarctation).

HYPOKALAEMIA

In any patient presenting with hypokalaemia it would be appropriate to check the following:
- electrolytes and renal function—to confirm hypokalaemia
- plasma bicarbonate and chloride—to check for metabolic alkalosis, usually a consequence of hyperaldosteronism (primary or secondary). A low plasma chloride would most commonly be explained by vomiting, which may be concealed
- urinary chloride—the diagnosis is hypokalaemia due to vomiting if the urinary chloride is very low
- urinary assay for diuretics and laxatives (in some cases).

Specific investigations

These will be guided by the clinical findings and results of routine testing.
- Renal or renovascular disease—consider 24-h urine collection for estimation of proteinuria and calculation of creatinine clearance; ultrasound to determine renal size and look for parenchymal abnormalities; renal artery imaging if renal artery stenosis (RAS) suspected (angiography—various techniques); renal biopsy if renal parenchymal disease is likely (see *Nephrology*, Sections 1.11, 2.5.1, 3.3 and 3.4).
- Primary hyperaldosteronism—which was the diagnosis in this case (see Section 2.2.3, p. 61).
- Cushing's syndrome—see Section 2.1.1, p. 47.
- Phaeochromocytoma—see Section 2.2.5, p. 65.

Management

Treatment is directed where possible at the underlying cause, with correction of hypertension and attention to target organ damage. Specific aspects of management relating to endocrine hypertension are outlined in the relevant sections of this module.

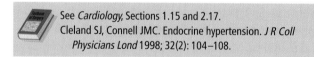

See *Cardiology*, Sections 1.15 and 2.17.
Cleland SJ, Connell JMC. Endocrine hypertension. *J R Coll Physicians Lond* 1998; 32(2): 104–108.

1.19 Hypertension and a neck swelling

Case history

A 32-year-old teacher is referred by his GP for investigation of a lump in the left side of his neck. He first noticed this 2 months earlier, following a sore throat. His past medical history is unremarkable apart from recently diagnosed hypertension (150/100), which has proved difficult to control with a β-blocker.

Clinical approach

The main concern is to exclude a sinister cause for the swelling. It would be unwise simply to attribute it to the recent sore throat: the patient and your defence union will not thank you if he subsequently presents with disseminated malignancy! Below is a list of the more common causes of neck swellings. It is also of concern that a relatively young man has hypertension, and that this seems resistant to treatment.

Causes of neck lumps
- Lipoma/sebaceous cyst
- Lymphadenopathy
- Thyroid pathology/thyroglossal cyst
- Pharyngeal pouch
- Muscle tumour/neuroma
- Aneurysm.

History of the presenting problem

Neck mass

Ask about the following if the details are not spontaneously forthcoming.
- When, where and how was the swelling first noticed?
- Has there been any change in its size?
- Has it been painful at any stage?
- Has he noticed lumps anywhere else?
- Enquire about local pressure symptoms, including difficulties with swallowing and breathing.

Then proceed to enquire about symptoms that might point to one of the causes listed above.
- Lymphadenopathy—many systemic disorders can present with localized lymphadenopathy. In particular, consider haematological malignancy, e.g. lymphoma, and enquire about classical B symptoms of fever, night sweats or weight loss. The history of sore throat may suggest recent infection including Epstein–Barr virus or cytomegalovirus (CMV). Pharyngeal and laryngeal malignancy can be associated with cervical lymphadenopathy, especially in smokers and heavy drinkers, but remember that even an infected bad tooth can cause lymphadenopathy (see *Infectious diseases*, Section 1.7; *Haematology*, Section 1.16; *Oncology*, Section 1.1).
- Thyroid disease—could the swelling be related to the thyroid gland? If so, ask about symptoms of hypo- or hyperthyroidism (see Section 2.3.1, p. 67).
- Pharyngeal pouch—has there been any difficulty swallowing? Has he ever coughed up bits of food some time after he has eaten them?

Hypertension

Enquire about the history of hypertension, considering secondary causes as discussed in Section 1.18, p. 40. Whilst much the commonest form of hypertension is 'essential', it is important not to assume this, especially in a young patient, and in this case there is particularly good reason to consider phaeochromocytoma, which could be associated with a concurrent neck mass in multiple endocrine neoplasia type 2 (MEN-2).

Relevant past history

Check for a family history of thyroid malignancy, severe unexplained hypertension or hypercalcaemia (for example manifesting as renal stones).

Examination

Overall impressions are important. Does the patient look well or cachetic? Perform a full physical examination looking for signs of systemic illness associated with lymphadenopathy (e.g. lymphoma).

Neck lump

> **Examination of a neck lump**
>
> Determine the following S features:
> - Site
> - Shape
> - Size
> - Surface
> - Smoothness
> - Solid/cyStic
> - Surroundings
> - pulSatility
> - tranSilluminability.

Thyroid

> **Examination of the thyroid gland**
>
> - Inspect from the front. Does the lump move on swallowing (give the patient a glass of water to help them to do this) or with tongue protrusion? The latter is suggestive of a thyroglossal cyst.
> - Stand behind the patient and palpate the gland assessing size, texture, mobility and smoothness. Is the lump solitary? Are there multiple nodules?
> - Check for tracheal displacement, tracheal narrowing (ask them to open their mouth and breathe in and out as fast as they can, listening for stridor as they do so), retrosternal extension (percuss over upper sternum) or a thyroid bruit.
> - Assess thyroid status (see Section 2.3, p. 67).
> If you have not already done so, check for lymphadenopathy.

Hypertension

Examine for features to suggest a secondary cause and for evidence of end organ damage as described in Section 1.18, p. 40.

Approach to investigation and management

Investigations

Regarding this man's hypertension, investigate as shown in Section 1.18, p. 40.

'Screening' investigations

Relating to the neck lump, the following are important:
- TFTs
- calcium and PTH (hyperparathyroidism)
- chest radiograph—look very carefully for lymphadenopathy (see Section 1.20, p. 45), masses or retrosternal goitre, and—if the latter is clinically suspected—request a flow volume loop to look for evidence of extrathoracic airway obstruction
- ultrasound scan—solid or cystic? Within the thyroid or outside of it? Relationship to blood vessels?

Specific investigations

These will be determined by clinical findings and those of the screening tests:
- lymphadenopathy—consider biopsy of an accessible node (ultrasound guided or surgical) if the cause is unclear
- thyroid—check thyroid autoantibodies and fasting calcitonin (medullary thyroid carcinoma); consider thyroid scintigraphy looking for hot or cold nodules; consider fine needle aspiration (FNA); a CT or MRI scan of the neck will help to delineate thyroid size, tumour extent and lymph node involvement (Fig. 19)
- pharyngeal pouch—cine swallow
- phaeochromocytoma—see Section 2.2.5, p. 65.

> **Imaging in phaeochromocytoma**
>
> Combined α- and β-adrenoceptor blockade is recommended prior to imaging with certain types of contrast agent if phaeochromocytoma has not been excluded (see Section 2.2.5, p. 65).

Management

- Management of hypertension is as discussed in Section 1.18, p. 41. See also *Cardiology*, Sections 1.15 and 2.17
- Lymphadenopathy is managed according to the underlying aetiology

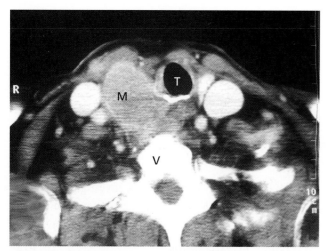

Fig. 19 Thyroid carcinoma. CT scan of the neck showing a large right-sided thyroid mass (M) displacing the trachea (T) to the left and extending posteriorly to the vertebral body (V).

- Thyroid nodules/carcinoma (see Section 2.3.3, p. 75; *Oncology*, Section 2.12)
- Phaeochromocytoma (see Section 2.2.5, p. 65)
- MEN-2 (see Section 2.7, p. 115).

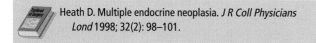

Heath D. Multiple endocrine neoplasia. *J R Coll Physicians Lond* 1998; 32(2): 98–101.

1.20 Tiredness, weight loss and amenorrhoea

Case history

A 42-year-old woman is referred by her GP with a 6-month history of tiredness and lethargy. Although 'routine bloods' were initially unremarkable, subsequent repeat thyroid function tests (TFTs) have shown a slightly elevated TSH with a low normal FT_4. Her husband reports that she has also lost a 'significant amount' of weight and her periods have stopped. More recently she has been troubled by nausea and vomiting.

Clinical approach

Although tiredness and lethargy are commonly reported symptoms of hypothyroidism, the relatively mild derangements of thyroid biochemistry reported here seem unlikely to account fully for the clinical picture. In particular, weight loss and oligomenorrhoea/amenorrhoea are more in keeping with thyroid hormone excess than deficiency. It is

therefore important to keep an open mind during the clinical assessment. Failure to do so, with treatment given simply on the basis of the biochemical abnormality, could lead to dire consequences.

History of the presenting problem

General

When did the woman last feel completely well? In retrospect, many patients can identify symptoms or signs in the past, which they ignored at the time or failed to associate with their current problem.

Tiredness and lethargy

Tiredness and lethargy are non-specific symptoms seen in the context of many different physical and psychological illnesses as well as in normal individuals, especially when overworked! See Section 1.14, p. 31 and Table 18, p. 32 for details of the approach to this problem. The most important issue to decide at the beginning is whether or not the tiredness and lethargy really amount to much more than might be expected given the woman's lifestyle.

- Does it affect her daily routine, e.g. is she still able to work/take exercise?
- Has the tiredness become progressively worse with time?
- Does she find it necessary to sleep during the day?

In this case a key point to note is the presence of other symptoms: weight loss, nausea and vomiting cannot simply be ascribed to 'overdoing it'.

Weight loss, nausea and vomiting

Important points are:
- How much weight has she lost and over what time period?
- Has this been associated with deliberate dieting or, alternatively, a loss of appetite?
- Confirm the timing of the onset of nausea and vomiting in relation to the weight loss.
- As a younger woman, did she have trouble with anorexia nervosa or bulimia? Has she ever made herself vomit?

Could a primarily gastrointestinal disease explain all of this woman's problems? Weight loss might be a reflection of reduced calorie intake, malabsorption or an underlying neoplastic process, whilst the development of anaemia could explain the tiredness and lethargy. Menstrual irregularities may accompany significant weight loss. Hence ask about appetite/dietary intake; abdominal pain/discomfort; altered bowel habit, e.g. frequency/constipation, blood, mucus. Further discussion of the clinical approach to weight loss with gastrointestinal symptoms can be found in *Gastroenterology*, Sections 1.10 and 1.11.

Oligomenorrhoea/amenorrhoea

Take a careful menstrual history. Ask about:
• age at menarche and regularity of cycle thereafter
• pregnancies and oral contraceptive use
• previous episodes of oligomenorrhoea/amenorrhoea or menorrhagia
• date of her last period, and whether it was 'lighter or heavier' than usual.

Further discussion on the clinical approach to amenorrhoea can be found in Sections 1.7, p. 18 and 1.8, p. 19.

Other features

This woman does not have symptoms confined to one organ system: how can this all be put together? Consider the following possibilities as you continue the history:
• malignancy and systemic disorders—weight loss and lethargy are common presenting features of malignancy (including lymphoma) and other systemic conditions (e.g. hepatitis, HIV-related disease). Ask about night sweats, lymphadenopathy and where appropriate assess risk factors (including sexual partners, intravenous drug use and previous blood transfusions—see *General clinical issues*, Section 2)
• depression/psychological illness—check for other physical manifestations of depression, including early morning wakening and constipation. Ask about mood and social circumstances
• thyroid disease—this has been suggested on the basis of the blood tests taken by the GP: check if there are any other symptoms to suggest thyroid dysfunction (Section 2.3, p. 67)
• Addison's disease—remember that many of the symptoms of Addison's disease are non-specific, often leading to considerable delay in its diagnosis. Tiredness, weakness, anorexia, weight loss and gastrointestinal disturbances are commonly reported. Menstrual disturbance may accompany the systemic upset
• pituitary disease—hypogonadotrophic hypogonadism and secondary adrenal insufficiency may complicate primary pituitary disease (e.g. non-functioning adenomas). Ask about headaches and visual disturbance (suggesting a local mass effect); galactorrhoea (hyperprolactinaemia—prolactinoma or stalk disconnection). Bear in mind, however, that the elevated TSH would be against coexistent central hypothyroidism
• DM—enquire about polyuria and polydipsia; prominent osmotic symptoms might be expected given the duration of illness and degree of systemic upset. Did the initial set of 'routine bloods' include a fasting glucose measurement?

Relevant past history

Is there is a personal or family history of organ-specific autoimmune disease, e.g. pernicious anaemia, vitiligo, thyroid disease (see Section 2.7, p. 115)? Ask about smoking and alcohol consumption.

Examination

General

Clearly, a thorough physical examination is necessary given the broad list of differential diagnoses. In addition, you will need to judge whether a psychological assessment is indicated (see *Psychiatry*, Section 1.6). Potentially there is much to be gleaned from general inspection of the patient, e.g:
• evidence of wasting/cachexia or anaemia
• the presence of a goitre
• generalized/palmar crease/buccal pigmentation
• abnormal mood/affect.

Gastrointestinal examination

Check specifically for:
• masses
• hepatosplenomegaly/lymphadenopathy (cervical, axillary and inguinal)
• abnormalities on rectal examination.

Examining a patient with non-specific or multisystem symptoms

Consider the following:
• thyroid disorders—look for hard evidence of thyroid disease, e.g. goitre, dysthyroid eye signs (hyperthyroidism), slow-relaxing reflexes (hypothyroidism)
• Addison's disease—check for pigmentation, low BP with a postural drop, scanty axillary/pubic hair
• pituitary disease—look for evidence of hypopituitarism (see Section 2.1.7, p. 57), visual field defects—especially a bitemporal hemianopia, galactorrhoea.

Approach to investigation and management

Investigations

Unless the diagnosis is apparent on the basis of the history and examination, a number of simple screening tests should be considered.

Screening tests

Dipstick urinalysis (renal disease). Full blood count with differential (anaemia; lymphopenia), urea and electrolytes

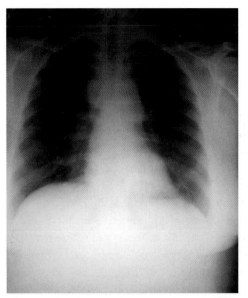

Fig. 20 Mediastinal lymphadenopathy. Chest radiograph demonstrating paratracheal lymphadenopathy in a patient with lymphoma.

Table 22 Primary and secondary adrenocortical insufficiency.

	Primary	Secondary
Cases (% of)	80%	20%
Aetiology	75% autoimmune	Hypothalamic–pituitary disease
ACTH	High	Low
Glucocorticoid	Deficient	Deficient
Mineralocorticoid	Deficient	Preserved
Na$^+$	Low	Low/normal
K$^+$	High	Normal
Treatment	Hydrocortisone and fludrocortisone	Hydrocortisone
Associations	Autoimmune polyglandular syndrome	Hypopituitarism

ACTH, adrenocorticotrophic hormone.

(Addison's disease, chronic renal impairment), fasting glucose, liver chemistry (malignancy, intrinsic liver disease) ESR and CRP (systemic disorders), FT$_4$ and TSH, prolactin. If malabsorption is a possibility check ferritin, folate, vitamin B$_{12}$, and antigliadin antibodies.

Chest radiograph—in addition to intrinsic lung disease, mediastinal lymphadenopathy may also be evident (Fig. 20).

Specific investigations

These will be dictated by the findings of screening tests:
- thyroid disease—see Section 2.3, p. 67
- Addison's disease—see Section 2.2.2, p. 59
- hypopituitarism—see Section 2.1.7, p. 57.

Table 22 outlines the main differences between primary and secondary adrenal insufficiency. This woman had primary adrenal failure.

Management

As always, management is directed at the underlying cause.

Addison's disease

The rules and regulations governing glucocorticoid and mineralocorticoid replacement in both the emergency and routine settings are discussed in detail in Section 2.2.2, p. 59. Note, as in this case, minor abnormalities of thyroid function may revert to normal with satisfactory steroid replacement.

Treat adrenal insufficiency before hypothyroidism

In both primary and secondary adrenal insufficiency, glucocorticoid replacement must be initiated before coexisting hypothyroidism is treated, to avoid the risk of precipitating a hypoadrenal crisis.

Hypopituitarism

In addition to treating the underlying cause, appropriate HRT should be instituted (see Section 2.1.7, p. 57).

For patients with secondary adrenocortical insufficiency, mineralocorticoid replacement is not necessary.

Communication

Patient education is extremely important for those with adrenal insufficiency. This woman will have to assume responsibility for a life-maintaining therapy that requires adjustment at times of stress and which may cause significant side-effects, particularly weight gain. Encouragement and advice will facilitate a return to her normal life style, including work and exercise. Those with Addison's disease and one or more of the other disorders associated with the autoimmune polyglandular syndrome type 2 (e.g. insulin-dependent diabetes or Hashimoto's thyroiditis—Section 2.7, p. 115) may be at risk of the particularly devastating complication of premature ovarian failure (POF). Depending on the patient it may be appropriate to discuss this, as she may decide not to defer having a family if the circumstances are otherwise appropriate.

See *Emergency medicine*, Section 1.20.
Oelkers W. Adrenal insufficiency. *N Engl J Med* 1996; 335: 1206–1212.

2 Diseases and treatments

2.1 Hypothalamic and pituitary diseases

2.1.1 CUSHING'S SYNDROME

This is the clinical disorder resulting from prolonged exposure to circulating supraphysiological levels of glucocorticoid.

Aetiology

 This is most easily thought of in terms of ACTH-dependent and ACTH-independent causes (Table 23). The term 'Cushing's disease' refers exclusively to those cases arising as a consequence of ACTH-secreting corticotroph adenomas of the pituitary gland, as described in 1932 by Harvey Cushing, an American neurosurgeon.

Clinical presentation

The clinical features of Cushing's syndrome have often been present for some time before the diagnosis is made. Patients may have been treated for individual components of the condition, for example obesity, hypertension or diabetes before the 'penny drops' and the diagnosis is considered. Women may present with oligomenorrhoea and infertility, whilst children can exhibit isolated growth failure.

Physical signs

Patients often exhibit many, if not all, of the classical signs (Fig. 21) of Cushing's syndrome, including:
- moon-like facies and plethora

Table 23 Aetiology of Cushing's syndrome.

Type	Example
ACTH-dependent	Pituitary adenoma (Cushing's disease) Ectopic ACTH secretion Ectopic CRH secretion (very rare)
ACTH-independent	Exogenous glucocorticoid administration Adrenal adenoma Adrenal carcinoma Nodular adrenal hyperplasia

ACTH, adrenocorticotrophic hormone; CRH, corticotrophin-releasing hormone.

- central (truncal) obesity ('orange on match-sticks')
- prominent supraclavicular fat pads and 'buffalo hump' (interscapular)
- acne, thin skin with easy bruising and purple striae (abdomen, thighs)
- hypertension
- muscle wasting and proximal myopathy
- hirsutism (but not in cases due to exogenous steroids which suppress adrenal androgen secretion)
- kyphoscoliosis due to osteoporosis
- psychiatric features, e.g. emotional lability, depression, psychosis.

 It is worth noting that in cases arising as a consequence of ectopic ACTH secretion, the clinical picture is often modified with wasting, cachexia and pigmentation more prominent, the latter reflecting very high circulating levels of ACTH.

Investigation

This should be approached in two stages:
- confirming the diagnosis
- defining the aetiology.

Confirming the diagnosis

Most centres use one or more of the following for screening purposes, with confirmation/further investigation of positive results.

Twenty-four hour urinary free cortisol (UFC) estimation

Two or more collections should be performed. Reference ranges vary between laboratories but in general levels >270 nmol per 24 h merit further investigation.

Overnight dexamethasone suppression test

One to two mg of dexamethasone at 11.00 pm, with 9.00 am cortisol the next day—normal response is complete suppression to <50 nmol/L. Note, however, that this test has a high false-positive rate (20–30%), such that some consider it to be of little use.

Low-dose dexamethasone suppression test

See Section 3.2.1, p. 121.

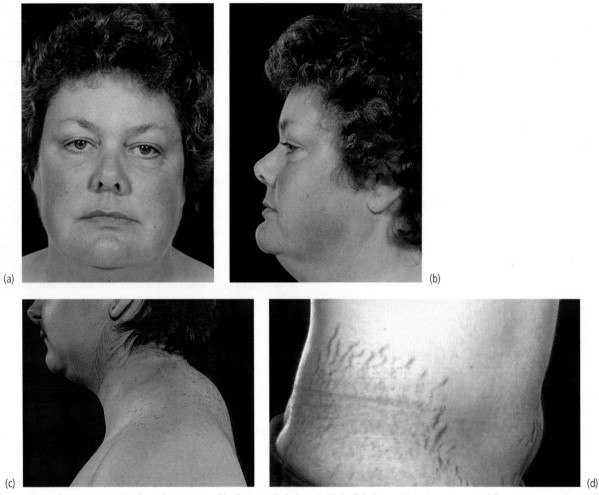

(a)　　　(b)

(c)　　　(d)

Fig. 21 Clinical features in Cushing's syndrome. Moon-like facies and plethora (a,b), buffalo hump (c) and purple striae (d).

Loss of diurnal cortisol variation

Measure 9.00 am and midnight cortisols—normal midnight cortisol, asleep, is <100 nmol/L.

Pseudo-Cushing's syndrome

A disorder mimicking Cushing's syndrome, and sometimes seen in the setting of excess alcohol consumption or severe endogenous depression, in which the overnight and low-dose dexamethasone suppression tests and UFC estimation can be abnormal. However, other indices (for example MCV, γ-GT) may suggest the underlying cause, and the cortisol response to insulin-induced hypoglycaemia (see Section 3.1.5, p. 119) is preserved, contrasting with the subnormal response typically seen in Cushing's syndrome. In addition, the low-dose dexamethasone suppression test followed at its conclusion by a corticotrophin-releasing hormone (CRH) test (see Section 3.1.2, p. 117) has been reported to reliably discriminate cases of pseudo-Cushing's from Cushing's disease.

Cyclical Cushing's syndrome

A rare variant in which hypercortisolism occurs periodically. Serial UFC collections may be required to establish the diagnosis.

Defining the aetiology

Once the diagnosis has been confirmed, tests are undertaken to establish the cause:

Plasma adrenocorticotrophic hormone

Distinguishes between ACTH-dependent and ACTH-independent causes.

ACTH-dependent cause

If an ACTH-dependent cause is suspected, consider the following.

HIGH-DOSE DEXAMETHASONE
SUPPRESSION TEST

See Section 3.2.2, p. 122.

CORTICOTROPHIN-RELEASING
HORMONE TEST

See Section 3.1.2, p. 117.

SELECTIVE VENOUS SAMPLING FOR ADRENOCORTICOTROPHIC HORMONE

If Cushing's disease seems likely, perform inferior petrosal sinus sampling, measuring ACTH before and after CRH stimulation. In a patient with Cushing's syndrome, an ACTH ratio of ≥2 between inferior petrosal and peripheral samples is indicative of a pituitary source of ACTH. Furthermore, a gradient between left and right petrosal sinuses of ≥2 can aid lateralization of an adenoma within the pituitary fossa.

IMAGING

Pituitary fossa

Although an adenoma can be identified in approximately 50% of patients with Cushing's disease, MRI/CT findings must be interpreted with care, since corticotroph adenomas may be too small to be detected, whilst pituitary incidentalomas (which are not clinically significant) are increasingly reported (up to 10% of normal individuals).

Chest and abdomen

Chest radiograph ± CT to look for ectopic sources of ACTH.

UREA AND ELECTROLYTES

Unprovoked hypokalaemia (i.e. in the absence of diuretics or other confounding factors) favours an ectopic source.

ACTH-independent cause

If an ACTH-independent cause is suspected, consider the following.

IMAGING

Adrenals

CT/MRI of adrenal glands—providing the patient is not receiving exogenous steroids, the main objective is to differentiate the possible adrenal causes, in particular adenoma (Fig. 22) and carcinoma.

Treatment

Initial treatment should aim to reduce circulating cortisol levels using drugs that block steroid biosynthesis, for example ketoconazole or metyrapone. Thereafter, specific treatment is directed at the source of hypercortisolism:
• pituitary adenoma—trans-sphenoidal adenomectomy or hemi-hypophysectomy. Radiotherapy may be required

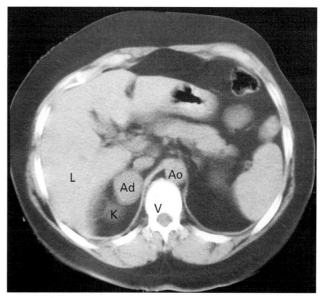

Fig. 22 Adrenal adenoma. CT scan showing a right-sided adrenal adenoma (Ad) in a patient with Cushing's syndrome. K, kidney; L, liver; Ao, aorta; V, vertebral body.

where surgical removal is incomplete or in patients judged unsuitable for surgery
• ectopic ACTH—surgical resection of tumour where possible
• adrenal tumour—surgical resection/debulking. For malignant tumours additional medical treatment is often necessary in the form of o,p,-DDD (mitotane), an adrenolytic agent
• exogenous corticosteroids—reduce dose or substitute steroid-sparing agents.

 Bilateral adrenalectomy is reserved for those patients in whom the primary source cannot be localized or when conventional treatment measures have failed. In Cushing's disease, however, this can be complicated by expansion of the corticotroph adenoma, leading to enhanced ACTH secretion, pigmentation and local problems due to tumour growth (so-called Nelson's syndrome). Pituitary irradiation may help to prevent this.

Prognosis

Untreated Cushing's syndrome is often fatal, predominantly as a consequence of the complications of sustained hypercortisolism, including hypertension, cardiovascular disease and susceptibility to infection. However, with modern surgical techniques, benign pituitary and adrenal tumours can often be removed in their entirety, thereby curing the patient.

 Orth DN. Cushing's syndrome. *N Engl J Med* 1995; 332: 791–803.
Trainer PJ, Besser M. *The Bart's Endocrine Protocols,* 1st edn. Churchill Livingstone, 1995.

2.1.2 ACROMEGALY

Acromegaly is the clinical disorder resulting from hyper-secretion of growth hormone (GH).

Aetiology/pathophysiology

The majority of cases are caused by a pituitary adenoma. Of these, 70–75% are macroadenomas (>1 cm in diameter) and 25–30% are microadenomas (<1 cm in diameter). A small number of cases have been reported in which acromegaly results from ectopic growth hormone-releasing hormone (GHRH) secretion. The growth-related aspects of this disorder are mediated by IGF-1 which is produced by the liver in response to GH, whilst GH itself has direct metabolic effects leading to insulin resistance (see *Physiology*, Section 5).

Epidemiology

The incidence of acromegaly is estimated at approximately 4–6 per million per year, with a prevalence of 40–70 per million. Patients are typically diagnosed in their early middle age, although the onset of symptoms often predates the diagnosis by 5–15 years.

Clinical presentation

The question of acromegaly is often first raised by a clinician, dentist or optometrist, who encourages the patient to seek advice for changes that they had attributed to 'ageing'. Commonly reported symptoms include:
• an increase in the size of the hands and feet (often noted as changes in ring and shoe size)
• coarsened facial features, altered bite and prominence of the jaw (prognathism)
• features of carpal tunnel syndrome
• snoring—reflecting sleep apnoea (which may be central or obstructive in aetiology)
• arthralgia
• sweating/oily skin
• thirst and polyuria (DM)
• local symptoms due to the space-occupying effects of a pituitary tumour, e.g. headache and visual disturbance
• amenorrhoea, loss of libido or erectile dysfunction secondary to hypogonadotrophic hypogonadism.

Physical signs

Many of the symptoms reported by the patient correlate with specific signs on examination, including evidence of large 'spade-like' hands and feet, prognathism and coarsened facial features (see Section 1.11, p. 25). In addition, hypertension is a common finding.

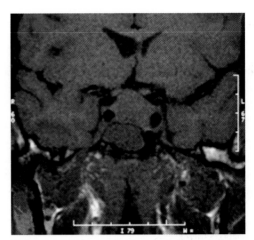

Fig. 23 Pituitary macroadenoma in acromegaly. Coronal pituitary MRI scan demonstrating a macroadenoma with suprasellar extension abutting the optic nerves and lateral spread to involve the cavernous sinuses.

 Careful examination of the visual fields is essential to check for evidence of a bitemporal hemianopia.

Investigation

Biochemical confirmation of the diagnosis is usually made using an oral glucose tolerance test (OGTT) (see Section 3.2.3, p. 122) in which GH levels show a paradoxical rise or failure to suppress in response to a glucose challenge. In addition, the IGF-1 concentration is typically elevated above the age-related normal range.

Once the diagnosis has been established, imaging of the pituitary fossa should be carried out (preferably by MRI—Fig. 23), and visual fields and visual acuity formally assessed. A full appraisal of anterior pituitary function is also necessary (see Section 2.1.7, p. 57). Remember that some GH-secreting tumours also produce prolactin.

Treatment

 Evidence suggests that if the mean GH level throughout the day can be reduced to less than 5 mU/L, the life expectancy of patients with acromegaly approximates that of the general population.

Surgery

The first-line treatment for acromegaly is usually surgery. In experienced hands, transsphenoidal adenomectomy offers a surgical cure rate of approximately 80% for microadenomas, but drops to less than 50% for macroadenomas. Recurrence rates are estimated at 2–7% over 5 years in patients originally considered to be 'cured' postoperatively.

Radiotherapy

Although not usually considered as first-line treatment, radiotherapy may be given if there is residual tumour postoperatively with persistent elevation of GH or if the patient is medically unfit for surgery.

Note that the beneficial effects of radiotherapy are delayed, with 50% of patients achieving adequate suppression of GH levels at 10 years. A similar proportion of patients at the same time point will have a degree of radiotherapy-induced hypopituitarism.

Medical therapy

The role of medical therapy in the management of acromegaly is evolving. Traditionally it has been used to supplement surgical treatment, as a 'holding exercise' in patients who have had radiotherapy, or as first-line treatment in patients who are unfit for surgery.

Somatostatin analogues

Somatostatin analogues (octreotide or longer acting preparations) are effective symptomatically in about 60% of patients, reducing GH concentrations to less than 5 mU/L in a similar proportion, and producing a significant reduction in tumour size in about 30% of patients. However, they are only available as injections, are expensive, and have gastrointestinal side effects, including an increased tendency to gallstone formation (requiring annual ultrasound assessment).

Dopamine agonists

Dopamine agonists (e.g. bromocriptine, cabergoline) only suppress GH levels to less than 10 mU/L in 10–20% of patients, athough they may be useful if the tumour cosecretes prolactin.

Growth hormone receptor antagonists

Clinical trials with GH receptor antagonists suggest that these agents are effective in blocking the actions of high circulating levels of GH.

Other risk factors

Aggressive treatment of other risk factors is beneficial, including hypertension, DM, dyslipidaemia and sleep apnoea. There is ongoing debate regarding the need for colonoscopic screening, an issue which has yet to be resolved. It is probably advisable in those with a family history of colon cancer.

A holistic approach

Other causes of morbidity should not be overlooked, with patients frequently requiring rheumatological/orthopaedic assessments, dental/maxillofacial opinions and psychological input or support to address problems of body image. They may find contact with The Pituitary Foundation helpful.

Follow-up

Following treatment, periodic MRI scans are required, together with assessment of visual fields, the GH–IGF-I axis, and anterior pituitary function.

Prognosis

The mortality of subjects with acromegaly has been estimated to be two to five times that of the general population, mainly due to an excess of cardiovascular, cerebrovascular and respiratory disease. Remember, the mortality rate approaches that of the general population if mean post-treatment GH levels are <5 mU/L.

Disease associations

Acromegaly may be associated with parathyroid and pancreatic tumours as part of the MEN-1 syndrome (see Section 2.7, p. 115).

Melmed S, Ho K, Klibanski A, Reichlin S, Thorner M. Recent advances in pathogenesis, diagnosis, and management of acromegaly. *J Clin Endocrinol Metab* 1995; 80: 3395–3402.

Melmed S, Jackson I, Kleinberg D, Klibanski A. Current treatment guidelines for acromegaly. *J Clin Endocrinol Metab* 1998; 83: 2646–2652.

2.1.3 HYPERPROLACTINAEMIA

Aetiology and pathophysiology

Varying degrees of hyperprolactinaemia are found in an array of physiological and pathological conditions (Table 24). Prolactin inhibits hypothalamic GnRH secretion and gonadal steroid production.

Epidemiology

Prolactin secreting adenomas are estimated to account for approximately one-third of all cases of secondary amenorrhoea in young women.

Table 24 Causes of hyperprolactinaemia.

Condition	Examples
Physiological	Pregnancy, lactation, postpartum
Idiopathic	—
Stress	Venepuncture (up to two-fold rise)
Drugs	Dopamine antagonists, e.g. phenothiazines, metoclopramide
Liver/renal disease	Cirrhosis, chronic renal impairment
Hypothalamic–pituitary disorders	Micro/macroprolactinoma, stalk disconnection syndrome (e.g. non-functioning tumour, infiltration)
Other endocrine disorders	Primary hypothyroidism (TRH is a trophic stimulus for prolactin release), PCOS

PCOS, polycystic ovarian syndrome; TRH, thyrotrophin-releasing hormone.

Clinical presentation

• Females typically present with oligomenorrhoea/amenorrhoea and/or galactorrhoea. Some are referred with infertility. On questioning, they may report symptoms of reduced libido and vaginal dryness with dyspareunia
• Males commonly present with larger tumours (macro-adenomas) causing local pressure effects (e.g. headache or visual disturbance), although reduced libido/potency, subfertility and galactorrhoea may occur.

Physical signs

Always examine for visual field defects (bitemporal hemianopia) and check for galactorrhoea. Signs of other underlying disorders (e.g. chronic liver or renal disease) may be present.

Investigation

Prolactin

The finding of an elevated prolactin level should be confirmed on at least one separate occasion.

 A prolactin concentration of >5000 mU/L usually indicates a prolactinoma, whilst values less than this may be seen with any of the other conditions shown in Table 24, including pituitary stalk compression.

Routine bloods

Check: renal, liver and thyroid function and carry out a pregnancy test if applicable. FSH, LH and E_2 may be useful in

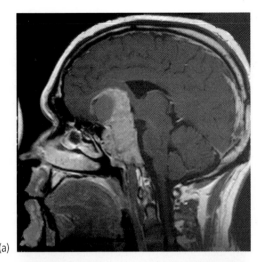

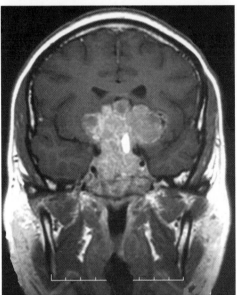

(a)

(b)

Fig. 24 Macroprolactinoma. Sagittal (a) and coronal (b) MRI scans demonstrating a massive macroprolactinoma. Note the heterogeneous appearance suggesting cystic components and areas of haemorrhage.

the differential diagnosis of oligomenorrhoea/amenorrhoea (see Section 2.4.1, p. 76).

Radiological imaging

Unless there is an obvious explanation for mild hyperprolactinaemia, an MRI (or CT) scan of the pituitary fossa is indicated in virtually all cases (Fig. 24). With modest hyperprolactinaemia, although a microadenoma may be identified, the principal objective of the scan is to exclude a tumour/infiltration causing disconnection hyperprolactinaemia.

Visual fields/pituitary function

Formal assessment of visual fields and anterior pituitary function (see Section 2.1.7, p. 57) may be indicated, depending on the clinical and MRI findings.

Differential diagnosis

The differential diagnosis of oligomenorrhoea/amenorrhoea is discussed in detail in Section 2.4.1, p. 76.

Treatment

Hyperprolactinaemia not associated with a pituitary tumour

- Drug treatment that is causing hyperprolactinaemia is sometimes amenable to change, in liaison with the original prescriber (often a psychiatrist)
- Women with unwanted postpartum galactorrhoea (and their partners) need to be advised to avoid nipple stimulation completely for a while, including 'checking to see if it is still happening'. Bromocriptine can be tried (see below), although some women find the benefit–side effect profile unfavourable and discontinue treatment
- Underlying renal or liver disease requires appropriate treatment
- Idiopathic hyperprolactinaemia—dopaminergic agonists are often effective in restoring prolactin levels to normal in symptomatic patients.

Hyperprolactinaemia caused by a pituitary tumour

Prolactinomas are unusual amongst pituitary tumours in that the primary treatment for both micro- and macroadenomas is medical (providing there is no immediate threat to vision). Dopaminergic agonists (e.g. bromocriptine) are often highly effective in shrinking tumours, relieving symptoms and preserving anterior pituitary function. Most microadenomas and approximately 75% of macroadenomas respond to bromocriptine therapy.

 The side effects of bromocriptine (including nausea, hypotension, nasal congestion and fatigue) can be minimized if the patient is started on a very low dose and advised to take the tablet with a snack at bedtime. Unfortunately, due to its short duration of action, bromocriptine requires frequent dosing. Longer-acting preparations (e.g. cabergoline and quinagolide) may therefore represent a more convenient option and appear to be better tolerated, although they are more expensive.

Microprolactinomas

Following normalization of prolactin, follow up is on an annual basis unless there is evidence of progression. Treatment may be withdrawn every 2–3 years to check for remission.

Macroprolactinomas

For those with macroprolactinomas, serial prolactin concentrations should be checked during the early stages of treatment and a repeat MRI scan performed to monitor the response to medical therapy. Additional bone protection measures (e.g. bisphosphonate treatment) may be necessary in patients whose prolactin concentration does not come down sufficiently to permit restoration of gonadal function. Remember that exogenous oestrogens should be avoided because of their potential trophic effect on the tumour. Surgical intervention (transsphenoidal adenomectomy) is generally preferred as second-line treatment. Radiotherapy is usually held in reserve for refractory tumours as it takes time to have an effect and often leads to hypopituitarism.

Non-functioning adenomas

Surgery is generally considered to be the treatment of choice (see Section 2.1.4, p. 54). For mid-range prolactin concentrations (4000–5000 mU/L), when it is difficult to distinguish between a prolactinoma and a non-functioning adenoma, a trial of bromocriptine may be considered to see if the tumour shrinks in response to medical therapy.

 The prolactin concentration is likely to come down with bromocriptine treatment in either case and therefore the size of the tumour must be monitored.

Contraception and pregnancy

- Women must be warned that they may get pregnant on starting treatment, even before they have a menstrual period. If they wish to defer pregnancy they should use barrier contraception, although the combined oral contraceptive pill is also safe for use in women with microadenomas. Those with microprolactinomas who do not wish to conceive do not need to take bromocriptine but should be on 'postmenopausal' HRT or other agents such as bisphosphonates to prevent osteoporosis. Again, contraceptive advice should be given.
- Bromocriptine is safe in pregnancy (there is less experience with cabergoline and quinagolide): patients with microadenomas are usually advised to discontinue treatment once pregnancy is confirmed, and are reassessed following cessation of breast-feeding. With macroadenomas some physicians recommend continuing bromocriptine throughout pregnancy, with avoidance of breast-feeding postpartum, in view of the small risk of clinically significant tumour expansion. Others withdraw bromocriptine but alert the patient to present immediately should they develop visual symptoms or a severe headache.

Complications

Prolonged oligomenorrhoea/amenorrhoea is associated with an increased risk of osteopaenia and osteoporosis.

Disease associations

Prolactinomas may rarely be associated with parathyroid and pancreatic tumours, e.g. MEN-1 (see Section 2.7, p. 115).

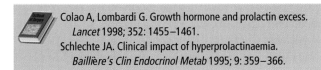

Colao A, Lombardi G. Growth hormone and prolactin excess. *Lancet* 1998; 352: 1455–1461.
Schlechte JA. Clinical impact of hyperprolactinaemia. *Baillière's Clin Endocrinol Metab* 1995; 9: 359–366.

2.1.4 NON-FUNCTIONING PITUITARY TUMOURS

Aetiology/pathophysiology

Non-functioning pituitary tumours ('chromophobe adenomas') are usually benign macroadenomas (>1 cm diameter).

Epidemiology

The incidence of non-functioning pituitary tumours is estimated at 10 per million per year.

Clinical presentation

Local pressure effects often result in a headache and visual disturbances. The patient may present with symptoms of hypopituitarism or hyperprolactinaemia due to pituitary stalk compression (fatigue, lack of well-being and hypogonadism). Alternatively, it may be an incidental finding following routine eye testing or a head scan for unrelated purposes.

Physical signs

It is important to check carefully for evidence of a bitemporal (sometimes only upper quandrantic) hemianopia. Features of hyperprolactinaemia may also be present (see Section 2.1.3, p. 51).

Investigation

A full assessment should include tests of anterior pituitary function (see Section 2.1.7, p. 57), an MRI scan of the pituitary fossa (Fig. 25), and formal tests of the patient's visual fields (Fig. 26) and visual acuity.

The serum prolactin result must be seen before surgery is considered in any patient with a suspected non-functioning tumour to exclude the possibility of a prolactinoma that would be amenable to medical therapy (see Section 2.1.3, p. 51).

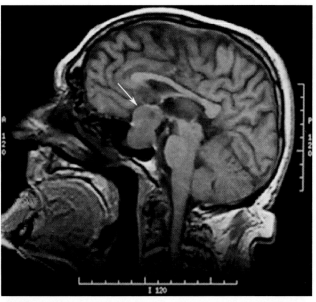

Fig. 25 Non-functioning tumour. Sagittal MRI scan showing a large non-functioning tumour arising from the pituitary fossa with suprasellar extension (arrow) in a 45-year-old man presenting with a bitemporal visual field defect.

Left   Right

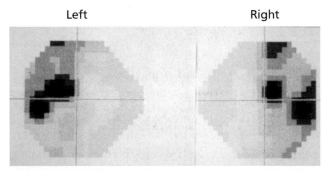

Fig. 26 Bitemporal visual field defect. Computerized perimetry provides accurate details regarding visual field loss. The shaded area centrally denotes the blind spot which is enlarged on the left side in this particular patient and is associated with a bitemporal field defect.

Differential diagnosis

The differential diagnosis includes other sellar or parasellar masses, including cysts, craniopharyngiomas, meningiomas, metastatic, infiltrative or granulomatous processes and lymphocytic hypophysitis.

Treatment

A non-functioning macroadenoma in a patient with pressure symptoms or signs, particularly loss of visual fields, requires urgent surgical debulking (transsphenoidal hypophysectomy or adenomectomy). Surgery may lead to partial recovery of anterior pituitary function. Postoperative radiotherapy should be considered if tumour removal is incomplete or subsequently if the tumour recurs.

If there are no pressure symptoms or signs, it may be acceptable in some cases (e.g. frail, elderly patients) to adopt an expectant approach. Either way, patients require serial MRI scans together with assessment of their visual fields, visual acuity and anterior pituitary function.

Complications

Operative complications include transient DI in 10–20% of patients, which may persist in 2–5%. Pituitary radiotherapy results in some degree of hypopituitarism in about 50% of patients after 20 years.

Prognosis

Hypopituitarism is associated with an increased mortality rate of at least twice the standardized mortality rate (see Section 2.1.7, p. 57).

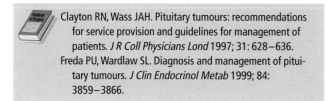

Clayton RN, Wass JAH. Pituitary tumours: recommendations for service provision and guidelines for management of patients. *J R Coll Physicians Lond* 1997; 31: 628–636.
Freda PU, Wardlaw SL. Diagnosis and management of pituitary tumours. *J Clin Endocrinol Metab* 1999; 84: 3859–3866.

2.1.5 PITUITARY APOPLEXY

Aetiology/pathophysiology

Pituitary apoplexy usually results from extensive infarction of a pituitary adenoma with haemorrhage. In ~50% of cases the event is spontaneous and the pathogenesis is not known. A quarter of all cases are associated with arterial hypertension and occasionally it is also seen following head trauma or dynamic testing of pituitary function.

Epidemiology

The incidence of clinical apoplexy in surgically treated pituitary adenomas has been reported to range from 0.6 to 9.0%. Although it can occur at any age, the mean age at presentation is 45 years.

Clinical presentation

Common

The classical presentation is with a sudden onset retro-orbital headache and visual disturbances, including reduced visual fields, visual acuity, photophobia and ophthalmoplegia (most commonly due to a unilateral 3rd nerve palsy). Symptoms may evolve over hours to days.

Uncommon

Occasionally the onset is more insidious with nausea and vomiting, meningism and an altered level of consciousness. Symptoms of hypopituitarism or hyperprolactinaemia, including chronic lethargy, reduced libido, oligomenorrhoea or amenorrhoea, impotence or galactorrhoea may also be present.

Physical signs

Common

Visual field defects and reduced visual acuity, together with ophthalmoplegia (3rd, 4th or 6th nerve palsies) are common. The conscious level may be reduced.

Rare

Signs of underlying pituitary disease (e.g. acromegaly) are occasionally present.

Investigation

An urgent MRI (or CT) scan of the pituitary fossa should be performed (Fig. 27). If this fails to demonstrate a pituitary haemorrhage, angiography may be necessary to exclude an intracranial aneurysm. There may be elevated numbers of red blood cells in the cerebrospinal fluid but, if the diagnosis of pituitary apoplexy is considered, a lumbar puncture is not advisable because of the risk of cerebral herniation. Blood samples for basic tests of anterior pituitary function should be taken, including cortisol, TFTs, prolactin, LH and FSH, and oestrogen or testosterone.

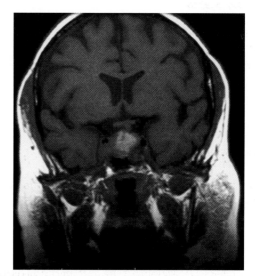

Fig. 27 Pituitary apoplexy. Coronal MRI scan demonstrating haemorrhage (high signal) within a pituitary adenoma in a patient who presented with acute onset of a severe headache and right 3rd and 6th cranial nerve palsies. Note the displacement of the pituitary stalk to the left.

Treatment

Emergency

> Once the diagnosis has been considered, anterior pituitary dysfunction must be assumed. Establish venous access (taking bloods for urea and electrolytes, glucose and cortisol) and give i.v. hydrocortisone (100 mg) immediately prior to establishing on regular replacement (see Section 2.1.7, p. 57). Fluid and electrolyte balance should be maintained.

Surgery

Urgent decompression is indicated if vision is severely affected. There is evidence that early surgery (within 1 week) improves both the visual and endocrine outcomes. In certain circumstances a conservative approach may be adopted, particularly if there is no progressive neuro-ophthalmic deficit, and/or if prolactin levels are very high (suggesting a prolactinoma that could be treated medically). However, this is associated with a risk of recurrent apoplexy.

Hormone replacement

A full endocrine evaluation should be made postoperatively, and appropriate HRT instituted with long-term follow up (see Section 2.1.7, p. 57).

Complications

Transient postoperative DI is common. The risks of permanent visual impairment and hypopituitarism are reduced by early surgery. Overall mortality rates are not known.

Gaillard RC. Pituitary gland emergencies. *Baillière's Clin Endocrinol Metab* 1992; 6: 57–75.

Randeva HS, Schoebel J, Byrne J, Esiri M, Adams CBT, Wass JAH. Classical pituitary apoplexy: clinical features, management and outcome. *Clin Endocrinol* 1999; 51: 181–186.

2.1.6 CRANIOPHARYNGIOMA

This tumour, typically comprising both solid and cystic components, arises between the pituitary and hypothalamus.

Aetiology/pathophysiology

The exact origin remains uncertain, but most probably arise within the pituitary stalk. Although histologically benign, local invasion is a frequent finding and many recur after surgery.

Epidemiology

Craniopharyngiomas are estimated to account for between 5 and 12% of all intracranial tumours in childhood and about 1% of brain tumours in adults. The peak incidence is distributed bimodally, with the majority of cases occurring between 5 and 14 years of age, but with a second smaller peak after 50 years of age.

Clinical presentation

Childhood

Although endocrine deficiencies are common, most go unrecognized for years and only come to attention when the child presents with symptoms of raised intracranial pressure (e.g. headache, nausea and vomiting) or visual disturbance due to the mass effect of an expanding tumour. GH deficiency is most common, leading to growth retardation.

In older children, there may be pubertal delay or arrest as a consequence of gonadotrophin deficiency. Features of hypothalamic dysfunction, including disturbance of appetite or thirst, somnolence and abnormal temperature regulation are sometimes seen.

Adulthood

Endocrine manifestations are a more common presenting feature in adulthood, although many cases exhibit symptoms of raised intracranial pressure.

Physical signs

Reduced visual acuity, and visual field defects as a consequence of chiasmal compression, together with papilloedema or optic atrophy (reflecting raised intracranial pressure) may be evident.

Investigation

Where possible, initial investigation of suspected cases should include:

Magnetic resonance imaging/computed tomography scan

MRI (or CT) scan of the pituitary fossa and hypothalamus. Craniopharyngiomas exhibit a distinctive appearance with mixed solid and cystic components, and heterogeneity of enhancement (Fig. 28). Intra- or suprasellar calcification is often evident on plain skull radiographs.

Ophthalmological review

To provide a baseline for monitoring the effects of treatment.

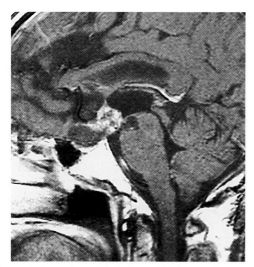

Fig. 28 Craniopharyngioma. Saggital MRI scan showing the typical appearances of a craniopharyngioma with mixed solid and cystic components, and heterogeneity of enhancement.

Assessment of hypothalamic–pituitary function

Nine am cortisol, thyroid function, prolactin, and paired urine and plasma osmolalities (with serum urea and electrolytes to look for evidence of DI). Approximately 80% of patients will have pituitary dysfunction at diagnosis.

Treatment

This is a rare condition and ideally patients should be referred to a centre with expertise in pituitary surgery.

Surgery

Fifty per cent of cases have evidence of hydrocephalus on initial imaging and one-third require urgent surgical decompression. Transcranial subfrontal surgery is usually required, although complete excision of the tumour is rare.

 Unless there is clear biochemical evidence to the contrary, assume that all cases have pituitary insufficiency and ensure that adequate steroid cover is given perioperatively (see Section 2.1.7, p. 59).

Postoperative

Short-term

Postoperative care will require combined endocrine, neurological, psychological and ophthalmological input. Since complete surgical resection is usually not feasible, adjunctive radiotherapy is often necessary and has been reported to reduce recurrence rates from 80 to 20%.

Long-term

Long-term follow up is required to detect and treat regrowth of the tumour and any hypothalamic-pituitary dysfunction. Patients and their carers may find contact with The Child Growth Foundation and The Pituitary Foundation useful.

Prognosis

Poor prognostic features include young age and presentation with hydrocephalus. Although non-malignant, craniopharyngiomas often have a worse outcome in childhood than other malignant cerebral tumours.

 Clayton RN, Wass JAH. Pituitary tumours: recommendations for service provision and guidelines for management of patients. *J R Coll Physicians Lond* 1997; 31: 628–636.
Lafferty AR, Chrousos GP. Pituitary tumours in children and adolescents. *J Clin Endocrinol Metab* 2000; 84: 4317–4323.

2.1.7 HYPOPITUITARISM AND HORMONE REPLACEMENT

Hypopituitarism denotes an insufficiency of one or more of the pituitary hormones.

Aetiology and pathophysiology

Destruction/compression of normal pituitary tissue or a reduction in the blood supply (including the hypothalamic-pituitary portal circulation) account for the majority of cases (Table 25).

 With pituitary tumours, the usual sequence in which pituitary hormone function is lost is:
- GH
- LH and FSH
- ACTH
- TSH.

Table 25 Aetiology of hypopituitarism.

Common	Pituitary/peri-pituitary tumours (or as a complication of treatment, including surgery and radiotherapy)
Rare	Pituitary haemorrhage or infarction (including pituitary apoplexy, Sheehan's syndrome and cranial arteritis)
	Pituitary infiltration (e.g. secondary malignancy, haemochromatosis, sarcoidosis, histiocytosis)
	Infection (e.g. tuberculosis)
	Empty sella syndrome
	Lymphocytic hypophysitis

Incidence

The incidence in adults is 8–10 per million per year.

Clinical presentation

This depends upon the aetiology, the degree of deficiency and the rapidity of onset. For example:
- chronic hypopituitarism (e.g. after pituitary radiotherapy) may present with general fatigue and a lack of well-being, symptoms of hypogonadism (sexual dysfunction, loss of libido, oligomenorrhoea/amenorrhoea) and possibly symptoms of hypothyroidism and hypoadrenalism
- GH deficiency may manifest as reduced exercise performance and quality of life
- Sheehan's syndrome (see Section 1.12, p. 27)
- pituitary apoplexy (see Section 2.1.5, p. 55).

Physical signs

The physical signs will generally be those of the primary hormone deficiency syndromes (e.g. hypothyroidism). Secondary hypoadrenalism may result in postural hypotension and loss of secondary sexual hair, but as the aetiology of the problem is pituitary hormone deficiency, it is not associated with hyperpigmentation. GH deficiency is associated with a reduction in lean body mass and an increase in fat mass (with an increased waist : hip ratio).

Investigation

Once hypopituitarism is suspected:
- complete biochemical assessment of pituitary function
- MRI (or CT) scan of the pituitary fossa
- formal testing of the patient's visual fields and acuity.

Anterior pituitary function

Growth hormone

Possible GH deficiency can be assessed using an insulin tolerance test (see Section 3.1.5, p. 119), which is usually supplemented with measurement of the IGF-1 level. The glucagon stimulation test provides a suitable alternative especially in children.

Gonadotrophins

In women with regular menses, who are not on the combined oral contraceptive pill, further tests are not necessary. Otherwise, LH, FSH and E_2 concentrations should be measured. In men, a testosterone concentration should be checked in conjunction with LH and FSH.

Adrenocorticotrophic hormone

Although a 9.00 am cortisol sample may be informative (e.g. if the value is very low), random measurements of ACTH and cortisol should generally not be used to screen for ACTH deficiency. Dynamic assessment of ACTH secretion (e.g. with an insulin tolerance test—Section 3.1.5, p. 119) is preferred.

Thyroid-stimulating hormone

Measurements of thyroxine (T_4) (ideally FT_4) and TSH are required to screen for TSH deficiency (see Section 3.3.1, p. 123).

Prolactin

Deficiency of prolactin is not clinically evident, except postpartum when it is associated with a failure of lactation. Hyperprolactinaemia is a more common finding in the setting of pituitary hormone deficiencies, reflecting stalk compression by an intrasellar mass/infiltration.

Posterior pituitary function

DI is unlikely if the urine output is less than 3 L in 24 h and the plasma sodium concentration is normal (see Section 1.3, p. 9). Glucocorticoid deficiency may mask DI because of the permissive effect of cortisol on water excretion. If necessary, a water deprivation test can be carried out (see Section 3.3.2, p. 124) after glucocorticoid replacement has been instituted.

Treatment

 Patients do not have to pay prescription charges for this type of HRT.

Hydrocortisone

- It is important to avoid the adverse side-effects of long-term treatment with supraphysiological doses of glucocorticoids. For most patients, 20 mg hydrocortisone daily is sufficient, divided into 15 mg on waking and 5 mg in the late afternoon, or 10 mg on waking, 5 mg at lunch time and 5 mg in the late afternoon. The adequacy of replacement can be assessed with a cortisol day curve.
- Patients must be given written advice about doubling or quadrupling their hydrocortisone dose if they are ill, and seeking medical help for intravenous therapy if they are unable to take their tablets. They should be given a steroid card and advised to purchase a 'Medic Alert' bracelet.

Thyroxine

The T_4 dose should be titrated to the FT_4 concentration (not the TSH level).

 Hydrocortisone replacement therapy, if indicated, must be instituted before T_4, to avoid the risk of precipitating a life-threatening hypoadrenal crisis.

Sex hormone replacement therapy

Both men and women require sex steroid replacement therapy to prevent osteoporosis.
• Women should be given cyclical oestrogen and progestogen or lower dose sequential HRT, especially if over the age of 35, until at least 50 years of age. Fertility treatment requires ovulation induction with gonadotrophins.
• Testosterone is usually replaced by intramuscular injections, implants or patches. Perform a rectal examination and check a prostate specific antigen (PSA) level before commencing treatment and periodically thereafter. Spermatogenesis requires specialist fertility treatment.

 Restoration of normal testosterone levels may not be welcomed by long-term hypogonadal males (or their partners!). In these circumstances consider alternative bone prophylaxis, e.g. with a bisphosphonate.

Growth hormone

GH replacement therapy is relatively expensive and remains controversial. Many clinicians only consider it in patients who are both biochemically and symptomatically GH deficient.

Recombinant human GH is self-administered by subcutaneous injection once a day. The dose is titrated to IGF-1 levels, against the age-related normal range.

Treatment may increase the patient's lean body mass, bone mineral density (BMD), exercise capacity and quality of life, and improve their lipid profile and insulin sensitivity. Effects on mortality are not yet known. The most common side effects of treatment are oedema and arthralgia, which respond to a reduction in dose. There is no evidence to suggest an increase in the risk of new tumour formation or recurrence of a previously treated pituitary tumour.

Antidiuretic hormone

Desmopressin acetate (DDAVP®) therapy is titrated to control symptoms of polyuria. It is typically administered intranasally or orally, with periodic monitoring of the serum sodium level to detect over replacement. Continuing polyuria and polydipsia suggest under replacement.

Prognosis

Hypopituitarism is said to be associated with reduced psychological well-being and a mortality rate which is at least twice the standardized mortality rate. This is a controversial area and the cause remains unclear, but may be related to periods of untreated hypogonadism, excessive glucocorticoid or T_4 therapy, inadequate glucocorticoid treatment in times of stress or GH deficiency.

 Lamberts SWJ, de Herder WW, van der Lely AJ. Pituitary insufficiency. *Lancet* 1998; 352: 127–134.
Monson JP. Adult growth hormone deficiency. *J R Coll Physicians Lond* 1998; 32: 19–22.
Vance ML. Hypopituitarism. *N Engl J Med* 1994; 330: 1651–1662.
Vance ML, Mauras N. Growth hormone therapy in adults and children. *N Engl J Med* 1999; 341: 1206–1216.

2.2 Adrenal disease

2.2.1 CUSHING'S SYNDROME

See Section 2.1.1, p. 47.

2.2.2 PRIMARY ADRENAL INSUFFICIENCY

Adrenocortical insufficiency may be:
• primary—arising as a consequence of destruction or dysfunction of the adrenal cortex, as described by Thomas Addison in 1855
• secondary—occurring secondary to deficient pituitary ACTH secretion (see Section 2.1.7, p. 57).

This section focuses on primary adrenal insufficiency and the clinical picture resulting from combined cortisol, aldosterone and adrenal androgen deficiency.

Aetiology

Although tuberculosis (TB) probably remains the commonest cause of primary adrenal insufficiency worldwide, in the UK more than 75% of cases are due to immune-mediated destruction of the adrenal glands, and may be associated with other autoimmune glandular hypofunction (see Section 2.7, p. 115).

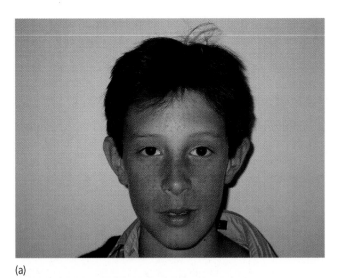
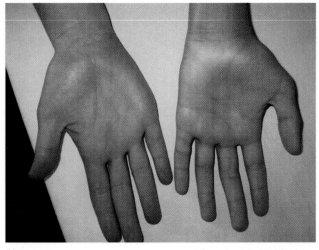

(a)   (b)

Fig. 29 Addison's disease. (a) Generalized hyperpigmentation of the skin and mucous membranes is one of the earliest manifestations of Addison's disease, and is increased in sun-exposed areas. (b) Increased pigmentation of the palmar creases (right), compared with an unaffected control subject (left).

 Aetiology of primary adrenocortical insufficiency

- Autoimmune
- Infection—TB, histoplasmosis
- Infiltration—metastatic malignancy/lymphoma; amyloidosis/sarcoidosis/haemochromatosis
- Iatrogenic—adrenalectomy; ketoconazole/metyrapone
- Adrenal haemorrhage
- CAH
- Adrenoleukodystrophy (rare X-linked disorder).

Epidemiology

Rare: prevalence <0.01% of the UK population, and with female : male ratio of approximately 3 : 1.

Clinical presentation

The clinical picture varies widely from the acutely ill patient in Addisonian crisis, to the relatively asymptomatic patient with pigmentation. When present, symptoms are often non-specific and the diagnosis is sometimes only made at *post mortem*, leading to its description as:

 'the unforgiving master of non-specificity and disguise' (CM Brosnan, NFC Gowing. *BMJ* 1996; 312: 1085–1087.)
Tiredness, weakness, dizziness, anorexia, weight loss and gastrointestinal disturbance are commonly reported. Some patients develop salt craving.

 Clinical features of acute adrenocortical insufficiency

- Fever
- Nausea and vomiting
- Weakness and impaired cognition
- Hypotension/shock
- Hypoglycaemia.

Physical signs

The more common clinical findings include:
- pigmentation—generalized (Fig. 29), palmar creases, scars, buccal mucosa
- postural hypotension
- loss of axillary and pubic hair in females (due to a lack of adrenal sex steroids).

Investigation

 In the acutely ill patient in whom you suspect adrenal insufficiency do not delay treatment:
- establish venous access (taking blood for urea and electrolytes, glucose and cortisol) and give i.v. hydrocortisone (100 mg) immediately
- set up a normal saline drip
- check blood glucose using a finger-prick sample.

In other non-emergency cases consider:

Urea, electrolytes and glucose

Note that the classical abnormalities—low sodium, high potassium, high urea and low glucose—are only seen in severe cases. Hypercalcaemia is occasionally reported.

Full blood count

Normochromic normocytic anaemia, neutropenia and eosinophilia are all recognized. The presence of macrocytosis should prompt consideration of possible coexistent pernicious anaemia.

Synacthen test

Short (see Section 3.1.1, p. 117) and long synacthen tests.

Short synacthen test—include a basal 9.00 am ACTH measurement (high in primary adrenal failure).

Autoantibodies

Check for adrenal, thyroid and intrinsic factor autoantibodies.

Chest radiograph/abdominal radiograph

Look for evidence of TB including adrenal calcification.

Thyroid-stimulating hormone and thyroxine

Ideally FT_4 should be used.

There may be concomitant thyroid dysfunction both in primary (autoimmune thyroid disease) and secondary (TSH deficiency) adrenal insufficiency. Note, however, that in Addison's disease, thyroid function abnormalities may revert to normal with satisfactory glucocorticoid replacement.

Treatment

Hypoadrenal crisis

Treat as above, and establish on regular 6-h intravenous intramuscular hydrocortisone (100 mg). Investigate and treat any precipitating cause.

Routine replacement

Hydrocortisone

Although most conveniently taken twice daily (e.g. 15 mg on waking and 5 mg in the late afternoon), thrice daily dosing (e.g. 10 mg on waking, 5 mg at midday and 5 mg in the late afternoon) probably achieves more physiological replacement. Adequacy can be checked with a cortisol day curve. The patient must be advised with regards steroid sick-day rules and carry a card/bracelet (see Section 2.1.7, p. 57) (Fig. 30).

Fludrocortisone

Start with 50–100 µg per day and adjust according to clinical status (postural hypotension, oedema, hypokalaemia) and/ or plasma renin activity (PRA). Usual maintenance is with 50–200 µg daily.

Adrenal androgens

Although not routinely given, evidence suggests that DHEAS may significantly improve well-being in individuals with primary adrenal insufficiency.

Thyroid hormone replacement should not be given until glucocorticoid replacement has been established due to the risk of precipitating an Addisonian crisis.

Prognosis

Providing hormone deficiency is adequately corrected, the underlying aetiology is often the most important determinant of outcome.

Arlt W, Callies F, van Vlijmen JC *et al.* Dehydroepiandrosterone replacement in women with adrenal insufficiency. *N Engl J Med* 1999; 341: 1013–1020.

Brosnan CM, Gowing NFC. *BMJ* 1996; 312: 1085–1087.

Hunt PJ, Gurnell EM, Huppert FA *et al.* Improvement in mood and fatigue following DHEA replacement in a randomized double blind trial in Addison's disease. *J Clin Endocrinol Metab* 2000; 85: 4650–4656.

Oelkers W. Adrenal insufficiency. *N Engl J Med* 1996; 335: 1206–1212.

2.2.3 PRIMARY HYPERALDOSTERONISM

Although rare, primary hyperaldosteronism is an important cause of hypertension in the young to middle-aged.

Aetiology

The majority of cases are due to benign aldosterone-producing adrenal adenomas, so-called Conn's syndrome. Other rarer causes are listed below.

Aetiology of primary hyperaldosteronism

• Conn's syndrome—benign aldosterone secreting adrenal adenoma
• Idiopathic hyperaldosteronism—commonly associated with bilateral adrenal hyperplasia
• Adrenal carcinoma
• Glucocorticoid remediable aldosteronism—an autosomal dominantly inherited disorder in which the 11 β-hydroxylase promoter is fused to the aldosterone synthase gene, allowing ACTH-sensitive production of aldosterone in the zona fasciculata.

Epidemiology

Accounts for 0.1% of all cases of hypertension, with a slight female excess.

Clinical presentation

Most cases come to light during investigation of hypertension or unexplained hypokalaemia. Non-specific symptoms including weakness, lassitude and polyuria may be reported, reflecting potassium depletion.

STEROID TREATMENT CARD

- Always carry this card with you and show it to anyone who treats you (for example a doctor, nurse, pharmacist or dentist). For one year after you stop the treatment, you must mention that you have taken steroids.

- If you become ill, or if you come into contact with anyone who has an infectious disease, consult your doctor promptly. If you have never had chickenpox, you should avoid close contact with people who have chickenpox or shingles. If you do come into contact with chickenpox, see your doctor urgently.

- Make sure that the information on the card is kept up to date.

I am a patient on STEROID treatment which must not be stopped suddenly

- If you have been taking this medicine for more than three weeks, the dose should be reduced gradually when you stop taking steroids unless your doctor says otherwise.

- Read the patient information leaflet given with the medicine.

Name	
Address	
Tel No	
GP	
Hospital	
Consultant	
Hospital No	

Date	Drug	Dose

Fig. 30 Steroid treatment card.

Physical signs

Mineralocorticoid excess *per se* is not associated with specific physical signs. The degree of hypertension is variable, ranging from mild to severe, although malignant/accelerated hypertension is exceptionally rare. There may be associated signs of target-organ damage, for example hypertensive retinopathy. Clinical evidence of oedema is rare.

Investigation

Prior to investigation:
- ensure satisfactory dietary sodium intake (>150 mmol per day)
- if antihypertensive treatment is necessary, use agents which do not interfere with the renin–angiotensin–aldosterone system, for example α-blockers.

Screening tests

Urea and electrolytes

The classical picture is one of hypokalaemic alkalosis. Serum sodium is usually normal to high.

Urinary potassium and sodium

Hypokalaemia is associated with inappropriate kaliuresis. Urinary sodium estimation ensures satisfactory dietary intake.

Plasma renin activity and aldosterone

PRA is suppressed in all cases of primary hyperaldosteronism, whilst aldosterone levels are elevated.

Determining the cause

Plasma renin activity and aldosterone

PLASMA RENIN ACTIVITY

In normal subjects, adoption of an upright posture for 4 h stimulates PRA when compared with resting supine levels. In patients with primary hyperaldosteronism, supine PRA is undetectable and remains suppressed despite ambulation.

ALDOSTERONE

Adrenal adenomas exhibit sensitivity to ACTH, and accordingly aldosterone levels fall in parallel with the circadian cortisol rhythm. By contrast, idiopathic hyperaldosteronism is associated with a lack of ACTH sensitivity, with aldosterone levels increasing on ambulation. Aldosterone values must therefore be interpreted in the context of the serum cortisol.

Computed tomography/magnetic resonance imaging of adrenals

Both techniques can be used to identify the cause of primary hyperaldosteronism (Fig. 31).

Labelled cholesterol scanning/selective venous sampling

Radionuclide scanning and/or selective venous sampling may be helpful in localizing adenomas that have not been clearly visualized with CT/MRI.

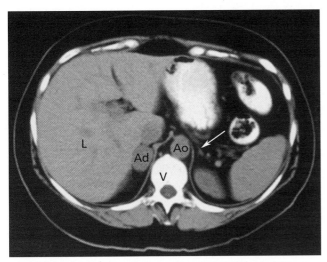

Fig. 31 Adrenal adenoma (Ad) in Conn's syndrome. Abdominal CT scan showing a right-sided adrenal adenoma in a patient with Conn's syndrome. The normal left adrenal gland (arrow) is just visible adjacent to the crus of the diaphragm. Ao, aorta; L, liver; V, vertebral body.

Treatment

Spironolactone is the medical treatment of choice because of its ability to block the action of aldosterone at the mineralocorticoid receptor. Treatment is titrated to normalize BP and restore normokalaemia.

Amiloride offers an alternative if spironolactone is poorly tolerated, and in some cases additional antihypertensive agents are required to control BP.

Thereafter, specific therapy is directed at the underlying cause:
• adrenal adenoma—unilateral adrenalectomy (some centres undertake this laparoscopically)
• idiopathic hyperaldosteronism—long-term spironolactone or amiloride.

Prognosis

Varies according to the underlying cause. For the majority of cases in whom an adenoma can be identified, excision removes the source of aldosterone but hypertensive end organ damage may be irreversible.

 Edwards CRW. Disorders of mineralocorticoid hormone secretion In: Grossman A (ed.). *Clinical Endocrinology*, 2nd edn, pp. 432–449. Oxford: Blackwell Science, 1998.
Mckenna TJ, Sequeira SJ, Heffernan A, Chambers J, Cunningham S. Diagnosis under random conditions of all disorders of the renin–angiotensin–aldosterone axis, including primary hyperaldosteronism. *J Clin Endocrinol Metab* 1991; 73: 952–957.

2.2.4 CONGENITAL ADRENAL HYPERPLASIA

Congenital adrenal hyperplasia (CAH) is not a single disease entity but encompasses several autosomal recessive disorders (arising as a consequence of inborn errors in adrenal cortical enzyme function), which result in varying degrees of impairment in the synthesis of cortisol and aldosterone.

Pathophysiology

The key stages in the steroid biosynthetic pathway are outlined in Fig. 32. Conversion of cholesterol to pregnenolone is the rate-limiting step and a major site of regulation by ACTH. 21-hydroxylase deficiency is the most common enzyme defect in CAH, with 11β-hydroxylase deficiency and 3β-hydroxysteroid dehydrogenase deficiency accounting for a relatively small number of cases.

Reduced cortisol synthesis is the common denominator, with consequent elevation of circulating ACTH levels further stimulating steroidogenesis. Precursors that cannot be metabolized by the deficient enzyme are then shunted down adjacent pathways, with the resulting clinical

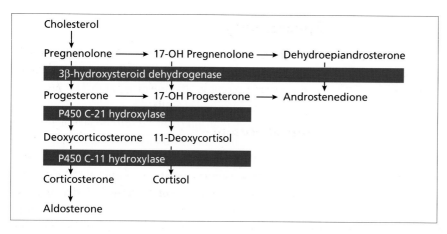

Cholesterol

Pregnenolone ⟶ 17-OH Pregnenolone ⟶ Dehydroepiandrosterone

3β-hydroxysteroid dehydrogenase

Progesterone ⟶ 17-OH Progesterone ⟶ Androstenedione

P450 C-21 hydroxylase

Deoxycorticosterone   11-Deoxycortisol

P450 C-11 hydroxylase

Corticosterone   Cortisol

Aldosterone

Fig. 32 Adrenal cortical steroid biosynthetic pathways.

phenotype reflecting both hormone deficiency (e.g. cortisol and aldosterone) and excess (e.g. androgens).

Epidemiology

The most common type, 21-hydroxylase deficiency, affects approximately 1 : 14 000 live births in Caucasians.

Clinical presentation/physical signs

Both 'classical' and 'non-classical' variants of CAH are recognized. The former denotes a more severe form, predominantly seen in the neonate or young child, whilst the latter is reserved for milder variants that often only come to light in adulthood. Table 26 indicates typical clinical features according to gender and age at presentation.

Investigation

Depending on the enzyme defect, different steroid precursors/androgens accumulate and can be measured in plasma. In practice most laboratories restrict screening to:
• 17α-hydroxyprogesterone (17-OHP)—this precursor accumulates in 21-hydroxylase deficiency. Its ability to discriminate from normal controls in mild cases is improved

following ACTH stimulation (Synacthen, 250 μg i.m.), which exaggerates the enzyme block (see Section 3.1.1, p. 117)
• testosterone, androstenedione and DHEAS—elevated in most cases
• plasma ACTH—elevated, although serum cortisol may be low or normal
• PRA—usually elevated in proportion to mineralocorticoid deficiency.

Screening

Identification of the genes encoding each of the enzymes involved in adrenal steroidogenesis permits screening for mutations using the polymerase chain reaction. For example, the 21-hydroxylase gene lies on chromosome 6 in close proximity to the major histocompatibility complex, and several common mutations have now been identified. One potential application of this technique is for prenatal diagnosis in families where there is already one affected child.

Treatment

Acute adrenal crisis

Episodes of acute adrenal insufficiency should be managed as outlined in Section 2.2.2, p. 59, with doses adjusted according to body weight/surface area in neonates.

Routine replacement

• Glucocorticoids inhibit ACTH release, restoring androgen levels to the normal range. Dose titration should be performed in relation to 17-OHP and adrenal androgen levels. In childhood this is particularly important as over treatment is associated with poor growth (through suppression of GH secretion). Standard steroid sick-day rules (see Section 2.1.7, p. 57) should be observed
• Mineralocorticoid replacement (fludrocortisone) is indicated in salt-wasting forms
• Plastic surgery may be required in cases with ambiguous external genitalia
• Psychological support is an important component of the long-term management of patients with CAH.

Table 26 Clinical presentations of congenital adrenal hyperplasia.*

Type	Age	Female	Male
Classical	Neonatal	Ambiguous genitalia Virilization Salt wasting	Salt wasting
	Childhood	—	Precocious puberty
Non-classical	Childhood Adulthood	Virilization Hirsutism Menstrual irregularities Infertility	Precocious puberty No specific symptoms

*Note that symptoms of cortisol deficiency are surprisingly rare, although hypoglycaemia is sometimes seen.

Prognosis

Salt-wasting forms are potentially life threatening if unrecognized. Once diagnosed, however, adequate treatment allows most individuals to lead a normal life and retain fertility.

Prevention

In those families in whom there is already one affected child with CAH, it is advisable to treat the mother with dexamethasone (which crosses the placenta) from the beginning of all subsequent pregnancies until chorionic villus sampling or amniocentesis is possible; the principal aim being the prevention of excessive fetal androgen production that would lead to virilization of an affected female fetus. If the fetus is found to be male or an unaffected female, treatment can be stopped.

Young MC, Hughes IA. Congenital adrenal hyperplasia. In: Grossman A (ed.). *Clinical Endocrinology*, 2nd edn, pp. 450–473. Oxford: Blackwell Science, 1998.

2.2.5 PHAEOCHROMOCYTOMA

In adults, phaeochromocytomas are known as the '10% tumour' reflecting approximately:
- 10% extra-adrenal
- 10% bilateral/multiple
- 10% malignant
- 10% familial.
  In childhood, a higher proportion are extra-adrenal and malignancy is more common.

Aetiology/pathophysiology

Originating from the chromaffin cells of the sympathetic nervous system, the majority of phaeochromocytomas arise within the adrenal medulla, with a smaller number derived from sympathetic ganglia. They commonly secrete norepinephrine (noradrenaline) and epinephrine (adrenaline), but in some cases significant amounts of dopamine may be released. As with many other endocrine tumours, the diagnosis of malignancy is often dependent upon evidence of local infiltration or distant spread, since histological appearances do not reliably distinguish benign from malignant tumours. Occasionally they occur in an inherited fashion, either in isolation or in the context of other syndromes, for example:
- MEN-2a and MEN-2b (see Section 2.7, p. 115)
- Von Hippel–Lindau syndrome (retinal and cerebellar haemangioblastomas)
- neurofibromatosis (Von Recklinghausen's disease).

Epidemiology

Rare, accounting for approximately 0.1% of all cases of hypertension. Many remain occult and are only diagnosed at *post mortem*.

Clinical presentation

Cases may come to light during the investigation of poorly controlled hypertension, when direct questioning reveals an array of other manifestations of catecholamine excess. These are frequently reported to occur in an episodic or paroxysmal fashion. Occasional cases present with pregnancy-associated hypertension, myocardial infarction, cardiac dysrhythmias or a dilated catecholamine cardiomyopathy.

Commonly reported symptoms of phaeochromocytoma

- Headache
- Sweating
- Palpitations/forceful heartbeat
- Anxiety
- Tremor
- Nausea and vomiting
- Chest and abdominal pain/dyspnoea.

Note that the triad of headache, sweating and palpitations is considered to be highly suggestive of a diagnosis of phaeochromocytoma.

Physical signs

Features of increased sympathetic activity are often present during a paroxysm. Hypertension may be sustained or episodic and approximately 50% of cases exhibit orthostatic hypotension (the latter reflecting intravascular depletion in response to long-standing hypertension).

Investigations

This should be approached in two stages:
- confirm catecholamine excess
- localize the tumour.

Confirm catecholamine excess

Urinary free catecholamines

Two 24-h urine collections for estimation of urinary free catecholamines (epinephrine [adrenaline], norepinephrine [noradrenaline] and dopamine) are considered to be the most sensitive screening method. Measurements of urinary catecholamine metabolites (metanephrines [MN]; vanillylmandelic acid [VMA]) are routinely performed in some centres, although both are associated with a significant false negative rate of detection.

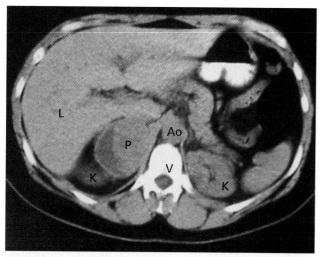

Fig. 33 Phaeochromocytoma. Abdominal CT scan showing a right-sided phaeochromocytoma (P). Ao, aorta; K, kidney; L, liver; V, vertebral body.

Plasma catecholamines

Useful in cases where paroxysms are infrequent and short-lived such that urinary estimations are within normal limits.

Localize the tumour

Computed tomography/magnetic resonance imaging

Both techniques are useful in localizing tumours to facilitate surgical removal (Fig. 33). A distinctive 'bright white' signal is seen on T2-weighted MRI.

 Intravenous injection of certain types of contrast media can precipitate pressor crises, and accordingly α- and β-blockade is recommended prior to examination with these agents.

Radioiodine-labelled metaiodobenzylguanidine scintigraphy

Meta-iodo-benzylguanidine (MIBG), which is taken up by chromaffin cells, is useful in localizing both adrenal and extra-adrenal tumours (Fig. 34). Pre-treating with potassium iodide blocks thyroidal uptake.

Differential diagnosis

Several conditions may present with features of sympathetic overactivity and thus mimic phaeochromocytoma (Table 8, p. 11).

Treatment

Medical therapy

Prior to considering surgical removal, medical treatment must be instituted with the aims of:

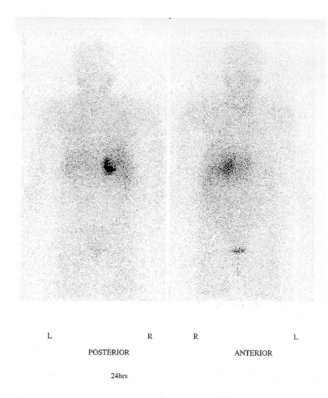

L R R L
POSTERIOR ANTERIOR

24hrs

Fig. 34 Phaeochromocytoma—Metaiodobenzylguanidine (MIBG) scan. The right-sided phaeochromocytoma shown in Fig. 33 demonstrates uptake of MIBG.

- ameliorating symptoms
- normalizing BP
- correcting intravascular depletion.

 β-Blockers must not be given to patients with suspected or proven phaeochromocytoma until α-blockade has been established, since there is a significant risk of precipitating a life-threatening hypertensive crisis due to unopposed α-adrenoceptor activity.

α-Blockade

The non-competitive α-antagonist phenoxybenzamine is the initial treatment of choice, with escalating dose titration (start with 10 mg twice daily and increase gradually until BP is normalized; most cases require 1–2 mg/kg per day in divided doses). The α_1-antagonist doxazosin provides an alternative for those intolerant of phenoxybenzamine.

β-Blockade

The non-selective agent propranolol (20–80 mg every 8 h) is generally preferred.

Surgical excision

Both traditional and laparoscopic approaches can be used for tumour removal.

Adjunctive therapy for malignant tumours

Options include:
- α-methylparatyrosine—which ameliorates symptoms through inhibition of tyrosine hydroxylase, the rate-limiting enzyme in the biosynthetic process
- radioiodine (^{131}I)-labelled MIBG—although large and repeated doses may be necessary.

Prognosis

Even those with malignant tumours frequently survive for many years. The extent of end organ damage is often a key factor in determining long-term outcome.

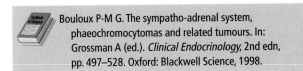

Bouloux P-M G. The sympatho-adrenal system, phaeochromocytomas and related tumours. In: Grossman A (ed.). *Clinical Endocrinology,* 2nd edn, pp. 497–528. Oxford: Blackwell Science, 1998.

2.3 Thyroid disease

2.3.1 HYPOTHYROIDISM

Hypothyroidism is the clinical syndrome that results from deficiency of the thyroid hormones T_4 and triiodothyronine (T_3).

Aetiology/pathogenesis

The causes of hypothyroidism are listed in Table 27. Iodine deficiency remains an important cause worldwide whilst, in the UK, autoimmune thyroid disease and previous treatment for thyrotoxicosis account for nearly 90% of cases.

The tendency for autoimmune thyroid disease (autoimmune hypothyroidism and Graves' disease) to run in families is strongly suggestive of a significant genetic component, although the nature of the interplay between genetic and environmental factors in their evolution remains to be elucidated.

Hashimoto's thyroiditis is characterized by lymphocytic infiltration of the gland and the presence of thyroid microsomal antibodies. Atrophic thyroiditis also appears to be immune mediated (with lymphocytic infiltration and microsomal antibodies) and is associated with other organ-specific autoimmune disorders.

Epidemiology

Hypothyroidism is common, with a prevalence of 1–2% in the general population. Females outnumber males by ~10 : 1. Congenital hypothyroidism occurs in 1 : 4000 live births in the UK.

Clinical presentation and physical signs

The classical presenting symptoms and associated physical signs of hypothyroidism are shown in Fig. 35.

Other presentations

Myxoedema coma

Patients with unsuspected or inadequately treated hypothyroidism are at risk of developing this rare but life-threatening condition. Coma may complicate an intercurrent illness (e.g. myocardial infarction, cerebrovascular accident, pneumonia) or be precipitated by certain drugs, particularly sedatives. Hypothermia is accompanied by bradycardia, hypotension, hypoglycaemia, hyponatraemia, hypoxia and hypercapnia.

Congenital hypothyroidism

The introduction of routine neonatal screening in the UK and other countries now permits the early diagnosis of this

Table 27 Aetiology of hypothyroidism.

Primary	Common	Autoimmune	Hashimoto's thyroiditis
			Atrophic thyroiditis (primary myxoedema)
		Previous treatment for thyrotoxicosis	Thyroidectomy
			Radioactive iodine
	Less common	Defects of hormone synthesis	Iodine deficiency (or excess)
			Drugs, e.g. antithyroid agents, lithium, amiodarone
			In-born errors of thyroid hormone synthesis
		Transient hypothyroidism	Subacute thyroiditis
			Postpartum thyroiditis
		Infiltration	e.g. tumour, amyloidosis
		Thyroid hypoplasia/agenesis	
Secondary	—	Hypothalamic or pituitary disease	

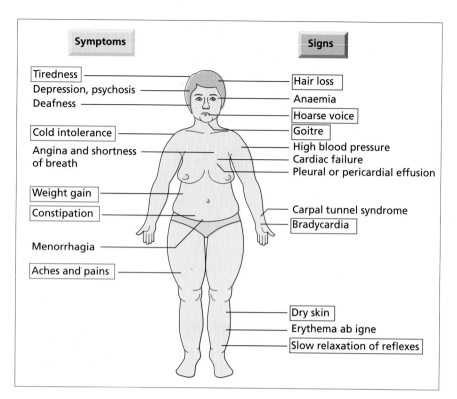

Fig. 35 Clinical features of hypothyroidism. The common symptoms and signs are shown in boxes.

condition which, if untreated, can lead to short stature, mental retardation and a characteristic puffy appearance of the face and hands (cretinism). It may arise in the setting of:
• placental transfer of TSH receptor-blocking antibodies from a mother with autoimmune thyroid disease
• maternal iodine deficiency or treatment with antithyroid agents during pregnancy
• thyroid hypoplasia/agenesis or inborn errors of thyroid hormone synthesis.

Subclinical hypothyroidism

It has been estimated that 10% or more of all females over the age of 50 are affected by this condition, which is characterized biochemically by normal FT_4 and FT_3 levels in the presence of a mildly elevated TSH. Although few report specific symptoms of hypothyroidism, hypercholesterolaemia and subtle cardiac abnormalities are recognized, which resolve following normalization of TSH with exogenous T_4.

Investigations

 It is important to have a low threshold for actively excluding hypothyroidism in 'at risk' groups, including those with:
• a goitre
• a history of autoimmune disease
• previously treated thyrotoxicosis
• a family history of thyroid disease.
And:
• in the elderly, in whom the symptoms of hypothyroidism may be mistaken for the normal ageing process.

Table 28 Abnormalities of thyroid function in various 'hypothyroid' states.

Condition	TSH	FT_4/FT_3
Primary hypothyroidism	↑↑	↓
Secondary hypothyroidism	↓ or →	↓
Subclinical hypothyroidism	↑	→
Sick euthyroidism	↓ or →	↓
Poor compliance with T_4 replacement	↑ or ↑↑	↓ or → or ↑

T_3, triiodothyronine; T_4, thyroxine; TSH, thyroid-stimulating hormone.

Thyroid function tests

Table 28 outlines the patterns of TFTs that are typically seen in various hypothyroid states (see Section 3.3.1, p. 123).

Anti-microsomal and anti-thyroglobulin antibodies

Anti-microsomal (formerly anti-thyroid peroxidase [anti-TPO]) and anti-thyroglobulin antibodies are commonly found in Hashimoto's thyroiditis and in atrophic hypothyroidism.

Full blood count

Hypothyroidism can be associated with anaemia (normocytic—impaired erythropoiesis; microcytic—menorrhagia, impaired iron absorption; macrocytic—B_{12} or folate deficiency).

Urea and electrolytes

Hyponatraemia may reflect increased ADH activity and reduced free water clearance or, if associated with hyperkalaemia, should prompt consideration of coexistent adrenal insufficiency.

Cholesterol and creatine kinase

Both serum cholesterol (total and LDL) and creatine kinase are typically elevated, indicating tissue hypothyroidism within liver and muscle, respectively.

Anterior pituitary function

A full assessment of pituitary function should be performed if secondary hypothyroidism is suspected.

Treatment

Myxoedema coma

Myxoedema coma is a medical emergency, with mortality in some series approaching 50%. Circulatory and ventilatory support are frequently required. Hypoglycaemia must be excluded, hypothermia corrected, and potential precipitating events sought and treated appropriately.

In the absence of clear evidence to the contrary, it is advisable to assume coexistent adrenal insufficiency and to give hydrocortisone 100 mg i.v. immediately. Steroid replacement should be continued until normal adrenal function has been demonstrated.

There is some debate as to the best method of starting thyroid hormone replacement. Levothyroxine (L-T$_4$) can be given as a single 500 µg bolus followed by a daily maintenance dose of 50–100 µg. Alternatively, it has been argued that liothyronine (L-T$_3$) should be the preferred mode of replacement due to its rapid onset of action and short half life, a typical starting dose being 5–10 µg every 6–8 h. Both can be administered by nasogastric tube or slow i.v. injection.

Long-term replacement

Although most cases of hypothyroidism require life-long replacement with L-T$_4$, occasionally thyroid dysfunction is transient, requiring only temporary treatment, e.g. subacute or postpartum thyroiditis. If this is suspected, then subsequent withdrawal of treatment should be considered, with repeat TFTs 4–6 weeks later.

The starting dose for L-T$_4$ is typically 50 µg per day. Assessment of adequacy of replacement and adjustments

to dose are made on the basis of clinical findings together with measurement of TSH and free thyroid hormone levels, initially checked at 6–8-week intervals. Once stabilized, the patient can be followed up by their GP with annual TFTs.

- The elderly and those with IHD may be particularly sensitive to T$_4$, and therefore lower starting doses should be used, e.g. 25 µg L-T$_4$ per day or on alternate days. If necessary, consider admission to hospital for supervision of replacement with ECG monitoring
- Always consider the possibility of coexistent adrenal insufficiency, and if in doubt exclude by formal testing (e.g. with short synacthen test) prior to initiating T$_4$ replacement.

- Remember that TSH should not be used to guide L-T$_4$ dose titration in cases of secondary hypothyroidism.
- It has been suggested that there may be some benefit in terms of cognitive function from combining L-T$_3$ with L-T$_4$ replacement to mimic the natural pattern of hormone release by the thyroid gland. This, however, is not routine practice.

Subclinical hypothyroidism

Management is mainly a matter of clinical judgement and each case should be dealt with on its own merits. Epidemiological evidence would suggest that there is high risk of progression to overt hypothyroidism in certain situations, e.g. in the presence of positive microsomal antibody titres. One suggested strategy for managing such cases is shown in Table 29.

Pregnancy

There is a higher incidence of stillbirths, miscarriages and congenital abnormalities in women with untreated hypothyroidism. In addition, evidence suggests that even mild hypothyroidism may have significant consequences

Table 29 Strategy for managing subclinical hypothyroidism.

If TSH >10 mU/L	Asymptomatic or symptomatic	Treat with T$_4$
If TSH 5–10 mU/L	Asymptomatic	Observe with repeat TFTs in 6 months
	Symptomatic	Treat with T$_4$
	Antibodies positive	Treat with T$_4$
	Abnormalities of lipids	Treat with T$_4$
	History of radioactive iodine or subtotal thyroidectomy	If asymptomatic, observe with repeat TFTs in 6 months, otherwise treat with T$_4$

T$_4$, thyroxine; TFTs, thyroid function tests; TSH, thyroid-stimulating hormone.

for the long-term intellectual development of the unborn child. Maintenance of TSH within normal limits is therefore important. Dose requirements for T_4 may increase by as much as 50–100%, especially during the latter stages of pregnancy. It is important to check TFTs in each trimester and adjust the dose of T_4 accordingly.

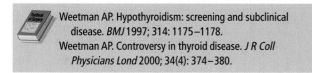

Weetman AP. Hypothyroidism: screening and subclinical disease. *BMJ* 1997; 314: 1175–1178.
Weetman AP. Controversy in thyroid disease. *J R Coll Physicians Lond* 2000; 34(4): 374–380.

2.3.2 THYROTOXICOSIS

Thyrotoxicosis is the clinical syndrome associated with raised levels of thyroid hormone (T_4 and/or T_3). Although usually the result of increased production of thyroid hormones (hyperthyroidism), it can also arise when stored hormone is released from a damaged gland (as in subacute thyroiditis) or when exogenous T_4 is taken in excess. Secondary hyperthyroidism due to increased TSH secretion is very rare and accounts for less than 1% of all cases.

Aetiology/pathophysiology

The causes of thyrotoxicosis are shown in Table 30.

Graves' disease

Approximately 15% of patients with Graves' disease have a close relative with the same condition, suggesting a

Table 30 Aetiology of thyrotoxicosis.

Primary	Common	Graves' disease
		Toxic multi-nodular goitre
	Less common	Toxic adenoma
		Postpartum thyroiditis
		Drug induced, e.g. amiodarone
		Over treatment with T_4
		Subacute thyroiditis
		Hyperthyroid phase of Hashimoto's thyroiditis ('Hashitoxicosis')
	Rare	Struma ovarii
		Metastatic differentiated follicular thyroid carcinoma
Secondary	Rare	TSH-secreting pituitary adenomas
		Trophoblastic tumours secreting hCG

hCG, human chorionic gonadotrophin; T_4, thyroxine; TSH, thyroid-stimulating hormone.

significant genetic component in the aetiology of this autoimmune disorder. Sensitization of T-lymphocytes to antigens within the thyroid gland leads to the production of autoantibodies (from activated B-lymphocytes), which are targeted against these antigens. The development of antibodies, which are capable of binding to and stimulating the TSH receptor, usually correlates with the appearance of thyrotoxic features.

In Graves' ophthalmopathy, infiltration of the extraocular muscles by mononuclear cells is accompanied by an accumulation of glycosaminoglycans (derived from orbital fibroblasts) which promote fluid retention, thereby effectively reducing the available space within the bony orbit.

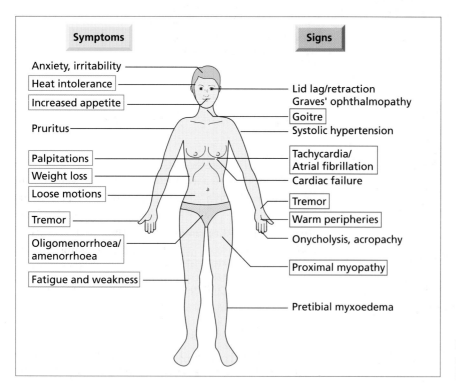

Fig. 36 Clinical features of thyrotoxicosis. The common symptoms and signs are shown in boxes.

This in turn leads to proptosis, ophthalmoplegia and the other features which typify Graves' eye disease (see below). A similar infiltrative process appears to underlie the skin lesion pretibial myxoedema.

Epidemiology

The prevalence of hyperthyroidism in the UK has been estimated at 1–2%, with an incidence of 3 per 1000 per year. Females are more commonly affected, especially in Graves' disease (5–10 : 1), with a peak age of onset in the 4th decade. By contrast, toxic multinodular goitre typically occurs in older patients (>50 years), often in the context of a long-standing non-toxic goitre.

Clinical presentation and physical signs

Figure 36 illustrates the common clinical features seen in thyrotoxicosis.

- Many of the manifestations of thyrotoxicosis reflect increased sensitivity to circulating catecholamines, e.g. tremor, sweating, anxiety. Included amongst these are the eye signs 'lid lag' and 'lid retraction', which are commonly found in thyrotoxicosis of any cause. By contrast, certain eye signs are specific to Graves' disease: proptosis, ophthalmoplegia, chemosis and periorbital oedema (Fig. 37). Interestingly, the development/progression of Graves' ophthalmopathy is independent of thyroid status, although there is a suggestion that it may be exacerbated if the TSH is allowed to rise during treatment. Overall only 3–5% of cases are classified as severe. The condition tends to be more pronounced in smokers
- Similarly, pretibial myxoedema is seen only in Graves' disease (Fig. 38).
  Table 31 summarizes the important differences between Graves' disease and toxic multinodular goitre.

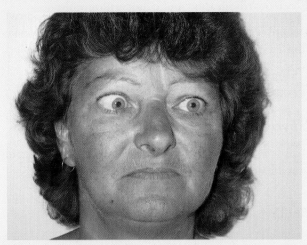

Fig. 37 Graves' ophthalmoplegia. Left 6th cranial nerve palsy in a patient with relapsed Graves' disease. Lid retraction is also evident.

(continued)

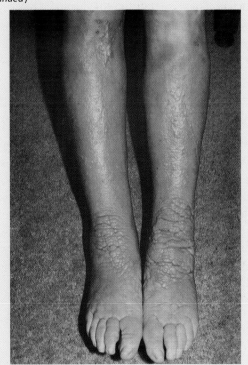

Fig. 38 Pretibial myxoedema.

Table 31 Clinical features of Graves' disease and toxic multi-nodular goitre.

	Graves' disease	Toxic multi-nodular goitre
Gender	Female ≫ male	Female > male
Peak age	20–40 years	>50 years
Goitre	Diffuse, smooth	Multi-nodular
Eye signs	Lid lag and lid retraction Graves' ophthalmopathy	Lid lag and lid retraction
Skin	Pre-tibial myxoedema	
Nails and fingers	Acropachy, onycholysis	
Autoantibodies	Usually present	Usually absent

Other presentations of thyrotoxicosis

The young and the old

Hyperactivity, increased linear growth and weight gain may occur in children with thyrotoxicosis. Older patients may present with apathy and depression or with symptoms of heart failure, angina or dysrhythmias (so-called apathetic hyperthyroidism). It is therefore important to exclude hyperthyroidism in any patient with atrial fibrillation or heart failure of undetermined aetiology.

Thyroid crisis

Patients with unrecognized thyrotoxicosis or severe poorly controlled disease are at risk of developing a potentially fatal thyroid crisis/storm. Precipitating factors include intercurrent illness, surgery, or ^{131}I therapy. Hyperpyrexia, profuse sweating, extreme restlessness, confusion, psychosis, dysrhythmias and features of heart failure are common manifestations. Left untreated, progression to shock, coma and death may occur within hours or days.

Pregnancy

The child of any mother with thyrotoxicosis during pregnancy, or with a previous history of thyrotoxicosis, is at risk of developing fetal or neonatal thyrotoxicosis, since thyroid stimulating antibodies may persist and cross the placenta from 26 weeks onwards.

Close monitoring is essential, especially in those who have previously received definitive treatment in the form of surgery or ^{131}I, and in whom high antibody titres may go undetected because of the lack of clinical signs in the mother. Monitoring of fetal heart rate, growth, and in some centres for evidence of a fetal goitre, may help to identify potential cases.

Neonatal thyrotoxicosis is more common than intrauterine thyrotoxicosis, often becoming clinically apparent 1–2 weeks after delivery. In either case, measurement of TSH receptor stimulating antibody titres in the mother and infant may help to predict the likelihood/severity of the disorder.

Thyroiditis

Several different forms of thyroiditis are recognized. In some cases there is accompanying thyrotoxicosis, reflecting destruction of thyroid follicles with resultant release of T_4 and T_3 into the bloodstream (e.g. subacute thyroiditis). This may be followed by a period of transient hypothyroidism, although in the case of postpartum thyroiditis up to 20% become permanently hypothyroid.

Differing types of thyroiditis

- Acute (suppurative)
- Subacute (de Quervain's or granulomatous thyroiditis)
- Drug induced (e.g. amiodarone)
- Autoimmune — chronic lymphocytic (Hashimoto's disease);
- Atrophic (primary myxoedema); postpartum; juvenile
- Riedel's thyroiditis
- Painless (non-postpartum).

Investigations

Thyroid function tests

- TSH is suppressed unless the cause is a TSH-secreting pituitary tumour

- FT_4 and/or FT_3 are raised. T_3 thyrotoxicosis (normal FT_4 in the presence of signs and symptoms, with a raised FT_3 and suppressed TSH) is more commonly associated with toxic adenoma.

Thyroid autoantibodies

- Microsomal antibodies (anti-TPO) are present in the majority of patients with autoimmune hyperthyroidism
- TSH receptor stimulating antibodies are usually detectable in Graves' disease. Measurement may be particularly helpful in certain situations, e.g. pregnancy (see above).

Radioisotope uptake scan

Radioisotope scans ([99m]technetium or ^{131}I) may be helpful in differentiating between the different causes of thyrotoxicosis (Fig. 39):
- in the absence of ophthalmopathy, uniform increased uptake suggests Graves' disease
- a patchy and irregular appearance is in keeping with toxic multi-nodular goitre
- a toxic adenoma will appear as a localized area of increased uptake with suppressed activity elsewhere
- in thyroiditis the uptake is typically low, although one should also keep in mind the possibility of iodine or T_4 ingestion.

Other investigations

Chest radiograph

Tracheal narrowing or deviation may be evident on a chest radiograph (Fig. 13, p. 31). Flow volume loops can help to confirm or exclude extra thoracic obstruction by moderate to large goitres.

Electrocardiography and echocardiography

If there is evidence of associated cardiac disease, e.g. atrial fibrillation.

Treatment

Thyroid crisis

This is a serious and potentially fatal disorder, requiring immediate emergency treatment:

Antithyroid drugs

Give carbimazole (CBZ) (20 mg orally) or propylthiouracil (PTU) (200 mg orally) immediately and continue every 6–8 h.

Addenbrooke's NHS Trust - Department of Nuclear Medicine

Anterior parallel   Anterior pinhole

(a)

Addenbrooke's NHS Trust - Department of Nuclear Medicine

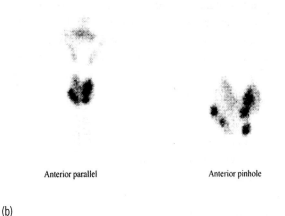

Anterior parallel   Anterior pinhole

(b)

Addenbrooke's NHS Trust - Department of Nuclear Medicine

Anterior parallel

(c)

Fig. 39 Thyroid isotope scans. Uptake of ^{99m}Technetium in Graves' disease (a), toxic multi-nodular goitre (b) and solitary toxic adenoma (c).

Iodide

Sodium iodide (1 g, i.e. 10 mL of 10% solution i.v. per 24 h) or saturated solution of potassium iodide (5 drops orally every 6 h) should be added 1 h later to prevent additional release of stored thyroid hormone.

 Iodide must not be started before organification has been blocked with an antithyroid drug due to the risk of providing further substrate for hormone synthesis.

Propranolol

One to 2 mg given slowly i.v. followed by 40–80 mg orally every 6–8 h, blocks many of the peripheral actions of T_3 and partially impairs conversion of T_4 to T_3. Verapamil (5–10 mg by slow i.v. injection) may be used if there is a history of asthma or evidence of severe cardiac failure.

Dexamethasone

Two mg orally (or i.v.) every 6–8 h helps to reduce peripheral conversion of T_4 to T_3.

Supportive measures

Oxygen therapy, intravenous fluids and active cooling (with cooling blankets and antipyretic agents—although avoid aspirin, which displaces thyroid hormone from thyroid-binding globulin) are usually required. Diuretics and digoxin may be indicated for cardiac failure. Chlorpromazine (50–100 mg i.m.) can be used safely as a sedative.

Short- and long-term treatment

β-Blockers

Non-selective β-blockers (e.g. propranolol 10–80 mg tds) are useful for symptomatic relief and rapid control of cardiac toxicity. They can usually be discontinued 3–4 weeks after commencing an antithyroid agent.

Antithyroid drugs

CBZ (40–60 mg per day in divided doses) will render most patients euthyroid within 3–4 weeks. Thereafter the dose can be reduced in a step-wise fashion to a maintenance level of 5–15 mg given once daily. Alternatively, after initial

73

blockade, a higher dose of CBZ (40 mg per day) can be maintained and T_4 replacement added in (starting with 50–100 µg per day) as part of a 'block replace' regimen, with the dose gradually titrated upwards if necessary. In Graves' disease, treatment is normally continued for 6–18 months. Following cessation of therapy, approximately 50% of patients will relapse.

 The effectiveness of treatment should be monitored clinically and biochemically with periodic measurement of FT_4 and/or free T_3. Remember that the TSH level often remains suppressed for several months after restoration of euthyroidism.

 Carbimazole

A number of patients are unable to tolerate CBZ, with rashes the most commonly reported adverse event (up to 5%). In a smaller number of cases (~0.5%), life-threatening agranulocytosis and/or thrombocytopaenia occur and require immediate cessation of therapy.

All patients placed on antithyroid drugs should be warned of this potentially serious side effect, and given written instructions advising them to immediately discontinue treatment and attend their GP or A&E department for a full blood count should they develop a sore throat or fever.

PTU represents an alternative to CBZ (with 200 mg of PTU equivalent to 20 mg of CBZ). It is often reserved for those unable to tolerate CBZ (although there are reports of agranulocytosis recurring after changing to PTU), and pregnancy (see below).

Radioiodine

[131]I offers a safe and effective means of treating thyrotoxicosis. [131]I is trapped and organified in the same manner as natural iodine but emits locally destructive beta particles that lead to cell damage and death over a period of several months. It is of particular use in the management of toxic multi-nodular goitre, toxic adenoma and relapsed Graves' disease. In some instances it is also preferred as first-line treatment for Graves' disease, e.g. in the elderly with cardiac disease.

Patients should be rendered euthyroid prior to treatment. It is necessary to stop antithyroid drugs 5–7 days before administration to allow uptake of the isotope. These should then be restarted 5–7 days after treatment and continued for a further 3 months. At this point residual thyroid status can be assessed. Long-term follow up is mandatory in all those treated with ^{131}I because of the high risk of subsequent hypothyroidism. Some regions operate thyroid registers that facilitate annual recall for TFTs in the community.

Table 32 Potential complications of thyroid surgery.

Early	Haemorrhage
	Vocal cord paresis
	Hypoparathyroidism
Late	Recurrent thyrotoxicosis
	Hypothyroidism

 • [131]I crosses the placenta and is therefore contraindicated in pregnancy which should also be avoided for at least 6 months after treatment
• There is ongoing controversy as to whether ^{131}I causes or worsens Graves' ophthalmopathy. Many centres avoid ^{131}I in moderate to severe eye disease, but permit treatment in mild cases under steroid cover (e.g. prednisolone 30–40 mg per day).

Surgery

Subtotal thyroidectomy is rarely the first-line treatment for uncomplicated thyrotoxicosis. It may be indicated, however, in the presence of:
• relapsing thyrotoxicosis
• compressive symptoms
• multiple allergies to medication or non-compliance with treatment
• toxic adenoma
• personal preference.

 Patients must be rendered euthyroid prior to surgery to minimize the risks of precipitating dysrhythmias during anaesthesia or of postoperative thyroid storm.

Table 32 outlines the potential complications of thyroid surgery.

Pregnancy

 Low TSH values are not uncommon in the first trimester. FT_4 levels are generally considered to be the best indicator of thyroid function during pregnancy.

 • [131]I therapy is contraindicated (as are radioisotope scans) and accordingly, treatment options are limited to antithyroid drugs or, in some cases, surgery during the second trimester
• PTU is preferred to CBZ during pregnancy and lactation because it crosses the placenta to a lesser extent and very little is found in breast milk. It is administered as a titration regimen
• Graves' disease often remits during pregnancy and some patients are able to come off antithyroid treatment completely. However, relapse is common, during the postnatal period
• TSH receptor antibody titres should be determined early in the third trimester to assess the risk of neonatal thyroid dysfunction.

Thyroiditis

Subacute, postpartum and painless thyroiditis are characterized by destruction of thyroid follicles with release of stored T_4 and T_3 into the circulation. In the thyrotoxic stage, β-blockers are the treatment of choice by virtue of their ability to relieve adrenergic symptoms. Antithyroid drugs are of little use. L-T_4 replacement may be required subsequently during the hypothyroid phase. The management of amiodarone-induced thyrotoxicosis is outlined in Section 1.14, p. 31.

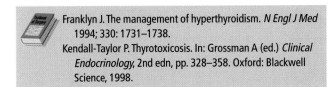

Franklyn J. The management of hyperthyroidism. *N Engl J Med* 1994; 330: 1731–1738.

Kendall-Taylor P. Thyrotoxicosis. In: Grossman A (ed.) *Clinical Endocrinology*, 2nd edn, pp. 328–358. Oxford: Blackwell Science, 1998.

2.3.3 THYROID NODULES AND GOITRE

The term 'goitre' denotes enlargement of the thyroid gland. It may be diffuse or nodular, simple or toxic, benign or malignant and physiological or pathological (Table 33).

Aetiology/pathogenesis

It is likely that an array of different factors interact to stimulate thyroid enlargement/nodule formation. For example, elevated TSH levels in hypothyroid states provide a strong trophic stimulus to the gland; similarly, antibodies directed against the TSH receptor may promote thyroid growth.

Epidemiology

Thyroid nodules and goitre are common; up to 8% of the population have palpable goitres and autopsy series report thyroid nodules in ~50% of people over the age of 40. Women are more commonly affected than men.

Clinical presentation

Many cases are noted incidentally, although there may be features of associated hypo- or hyperthyroidism. Occasionally, thyroid enlargement leads to local pressure symptoms, e.g. difficulty in breathing (with stridor) or swallowing.

Physical signs

An approach to the examination of the thyroid gland is outlined in Section 1.19, p. 42. Remember to check for the presence of lymphadenopathy—enlarged lymph nodes in the cervical chain may be a sinister feature when associated with a thyroid nodule.

Investigations

Blood tests

Thyroid function tests

FT_4, FT_3 and TSH should be checked to exclude overt thyroid dysfunction.

 Apparent subclinical hyperthyroidism (normal free thyroid hormone levels in the presence of a suppressed TSH) is a relatively common finding in clinically euthyroid patients with nodule(s) or goitre; it does not require specific antithyroid drug treatment.

Thyroid antibodies

The demonstration of positive thyroid antibody titres (microsomal, thyroglobulin) may support your suspicions of underlying autoimmune disease. However, it does not exclude coexistent pathology, including malignancy.

Calcitonin

Measurement of basal and stimulated calcitonin levels (see Section 3.1.6, p. 120) is reserved for cases where medullary thyroid carcinoma is suspected (e.g. in those with a family history of MEN-2) (see Section 2.7, p. 115).

Table 33 Classification of goitre and thyroid nodules.

	Type	Cause
Diffuse goitre	Physiological	Puberty
		Pregnancy
	Autoimmune	Graves' disease
		Hashimoto's thyroiditis
	Thyroiditis	Subacute (de Quervain's)
		Reidel's disease
	Iodine deficiency (endogenous goitre)	—
	Dyshormonogenesis	—
	Goitrogens	Antithyroid drugs
		Lithium
		Iodine excess
Nodular goitre	Multi-nodular goitre	Toxic
		Non-toxic
	Solitary nodule	Toxic adenoma
		Benign nodule
		Malignant nodule
		Lymphoma
		Metastasis
	Infiltration (rare)	Tuberculosis
		Sarcoidosis

Thyroglobulin

Although thyroglobulin estimation serves as a valuable tumour marker in individuals with differentiated thyroid carcinoma who have undergone completion thyroidectomy, it is of little use in the screening of newly presenting nodules/goitre, since levels are also elevated in several benign conditions.

Imaging

Plain radiographs/computed tomography

Radiographs of the chest and thoracic inlet may demonstrate retrosternal extension of a goitre and/or compression of surrounding structures (Fig. 13, p. 31), which can be confirmed on CT examination. Flow-volume loop studies should be considered in such cases.

Ultrasonography

Although ultrasound is helpful in distinguishing between solid, cystic or mixed (solid and cystic) nodules, it cannot reliably differentiate between benign and malignant lesions.

^{99m}Technetium scintigraphy

Radioisotope scans are not routinely used in the investigation of thyroid nodules since the identification of a 'cold' or 'hot' lesion does not necessarily correlate with the presence of a malignant or benign lesion, respectively.

- Less than 20% of cold nodules are malignant. The remainder are benign (colloid nodules, Hashimoto's thyroiditis, haemorrhage)
- The presence of a 'warm' or 'hot' nodule does not exclude malignancy
- On ultrasound, a solid nodule is more likely to be malignant than a cystic lesion. However, the majority of solid nodules are benign, whilst some cystic lesions are malignant.

Fine needle aspiration (FNA) biopsy/ ultrasound guided biopsy

Due to the lack of sensitivity and specificity of clinical examination and routine radiology in the differentiation of benign from malignant solitary/dominant thyroid nodules, FNA biopsy is the first-line investigation in such cases. Results are typically reported as either:
- non-diagnostic (indicating a need for repeat aspiration)
- benign
- suspicious
- malignant.

The latter two groups should be referred for surgical management, whilst those with benign cytology can be observed. The identification of a follicular lesion merits special mention, however, since follicular adenomas cannot be distinguished from carcinomas on FNA biopsy and accordingly all require referral for surgery.

Treatment

Wherever possible, the underlying condition should be treated appropriately, e.g. T_4 replacement in hypothyroidism associated with Hashimoto's thyroiditis; thyroidectomy for suspicious or frankly malignant nodules. Surgery may also be indicated for single benign nodules or non-toxic multi-nodular goitre associated with local pressure effects, although ^{131}I may be equally as effective in the long term.

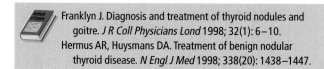
Franklyn J. Diagnosis and treatment of thyroid nodules and goitre. *J R Coll Physicians Lond* 1998; 32(1): 6–10.
Hermus AR, Huysmans DA. Treatment of benign nodular thyroid disease. *N Engl J Med* 1998; 338(20): 1438–1447.

2.3.4 THYROID MALIGNANCY

Thyroid malignancy represents the commonest of the endocrine cancers. Although several mutations have been described in various protooncogenes (e.g. the *PTC/RET* mutation in some cases of papillary carcinoma) and tumour suppressor genes (e.g. p53 mutations in anaplastic carcinoma), considerable work remains to be done to understand the molecular basis for thyroid carcinoma. Table 34 outlines the important clinical aspects of this disorder. See also *Oncology*, Section 2.12.

2.4 Reproductive diseases

2.4.1 OLIGOMENORRHOEA/ AMENORRHOEA AND PREMATURE MENOPAUSE

Amenorrhoea is traditionally subdivided into:
- primary amenorrhoea: lack of menses by the age of 16
- secondary amenorrhoea: absence of menstrual periods for 6 months or more after cyclical menses have been established.
Oligomenorrhoea indicates lighter/irregular periods.

Aetiology/pathophysiology

In practice, there is considerable overlap between primary and secondary amenorrhoea, as a number of conditions can give rise to either (Table 35). A small number of disorders are, however, specifically associated with primary

Table 34 Clinical aspects of thyroid malignancy.

Type of thyroid malignancy	Epidemiology	Clinical features/spread/metastases	Treatment/prognosis
Papillary	• ~70% of all cases • ♂:♀ ~ 1:3 • Peak incidence during the 4th decade of life	Considered to be the slowest growing of the thyroid cancers. Although local spread to cervical lymph nodes is not uncommon at presentation, distant metastases are rare	Total thyroidectomy is recommended for all but the smallest of tumours, and is followed by an ablative dose of radioactive iodine. This in turn is followed by life-long suppressive T_4 therapy. In these circumstances thyroglobulin acts as a useful tumour marker. Cancer-related death occurs in only ~10% of cases during 20 years follow up
Follicular	• ~15% of all cases • ♂:♀ ~ 1:2.5 • Peak incidence during the 5th decade of life	More aggressive than papillary carcinoma. Spread may occur by local invasion of lymph nodes or by blood vessel invasion with distant metastases to lung and bone	Follicular carcinoma is treated along the same lines as papillary carcinoma. However, cancer-related deaths occur in a higher proportion of patients (20–60%) during 20 years follow up
Anaplastic	• <10% of all cases • ♂:♀ ~ 1:1 • Peak incidence between 65 and 70 years of age	An aggressive form of thyroid cancer, which typically presents with a painful rapidly expanding thyroid mass	Despite combined treatment with surgery, radiotherapy and in some cases chemotherapy, the prognosis is poor, with few patients surviving more than 6–8 months
MTC	• < 5% of all cases • ♂:♀ ~ 1:1 • Sporadic MTC has a peak incidence in the 4th–5th decades, whilst hereditary MTC is often detected at a much earlier age	More aggressive than papillary or follicular carcinoma, but less so than anaplastic tumours. Locally invasive with distant spread via lymphatics and blood. Associated with the MEN-2 syndromes	Total thyroidectomy may be curative in the early stages, hence the rationale for screening relatives of affected individuals in MEN kindreds. Radiotherapy and chemotherapy are usually of little benefit. Long-term survival is variable
Lymphoma	<1% of all cases	May arise as a primary in the thyroid or as part of a generalized lymphoma	Variable prognosis and response to radiotherapy

MEN, multiple endocrine neoplasia; MEN-2, multiple endocrine neoplasia type 2; MTC, medullary thyroid carcinoma; T_4, thyroxine.

Table 35 Causes of amenorrhoea.

Physiological	Pubertal delay Pregnancy Lactation Post-menopausal
Pathological	PCOS Hypothalamic–pituitary dysfunction (including excessive weight loss or exercise, stress, pituitary tumours/infiltration, hyperprolactinaemia) Turner's syndrome Premature ovarian failure (POF) Congenital adrenal hyperplasia Adrenal/ovarian neoplasms Congenital anomalies of the female reproductive tract

PCOS, polycystic ovarian syndrome.

amenorrhoea, including anatomical defects of the female reproductive tract and Turner's syndrome.

 Most clinicians agree that 'post-pill amenorrhoea' does not exist, and that an underlying cause should be sought in such cases.

Clinical presentation

Common

- Oligomenorrhoea/amenorrhoea
- Impaired fertility
- Hirsutism or acne.

Uncommon

Menopausal symptoms including:
- hot flushes
- night sweats
- vaginal dryness ± dyspareunia.

Rare

If there is a space-occupying pituitary lesion:
- visual symptoms
- headache
- features of other pituitary hormone deficiency or excess.

Physical signs

Common

- Extremes of BMI (>30 or <20 kg/m²)
- Mild hirsutism or acne.

Rare

- Virilization (marked hirsutism, muscle development in a male pattern, clitoromegaly)
- Bitemporal hemianopia (suggestive of a pituitary tumour).

Investigation

 • Patients should be fully evaluated at initial presentation: subfertility is always an urgent concern, and prolonged low oestrogen levels may lead to osteopaenia and osteoporosis. However, before embarking on more complex investigations the possibility of pregnancy must be considered to prevent embarrassment for all concerned at a later date!

Once pregnancy has been excluded, baseline investigations should include measurement of:
- gonadotrophins—FSH and LH
- E_2
- prolactin.

Together with the clinical features, these preliminary screening tests will guide subsequent investigations (Table 36), which may include:
- TFTs (ideally FT_4 and TSH to distinguish primary and secondary thyroid dysfunction)
- dynamic assessment of pituitary reserve, e.g. insulin tolerance test (see Section 3.1.5, p. 119)
- testosterone and DHEAS (if there are any signs of androgen excess)
- 17-OHP (late-onset CAH may present in adulthood with oligomenorrhoea) (see Section 2.2.4, p. 63)
- a Provera® (medroxyprogesterone) withdrawal test. In non-pregnant patients, Provera® at a dose of 10 mg daily is administered for 5 days. If a withdrawal bleed occurs within 10 days, the endometrium must have been exposed to oestrogen, and it is generally accepted that oestrogen levels are sufficient to protect the patient's bones, even if she is amenorrhoeic
- a mid-luteal phase (day 21) progesterone. In menstruating patients, a level of more than 30 nmol/L suggests that ovulation has occurred during that cycle
- karyotype analysis (Turner's syndrome)
- radiological imaging of the pituitary, adrenals or ovaries, depending on the biochemical pattern of results.

Treatment

General

Specific treatment should be directed at the underlying disorder. Weight adjustment may be effective in hypo-gonadotrophic hypogonadism and PCOS but is often very difficult for the patient to achieve.

Osteoporosis

Oestrogen therapy (with a cyclical progestogen unless the patient has had a hysterectomy) is indicated to prevent osteoporosis if the Provera® test is negative. This can be given in the form of postmenopausal HRT (which would not prevent conception, however unlikely), or the combined oral contraceptive pill.

Fertility

Hypogonadotrophic hypogonadism may respond to specialist treatment with gonadotrophins and GnRH. In women with POF, in-vitro fertilization using a donated oocyte is the only option.

Complications

- Osteopaenia, with the subsequent risk of osteoporotic fractures, due to oestrogen deficiency
- Psychological problems linked to impaired fertility or hirsutism.

Disease associations

POF may be associated with other autoimmune endocrine disorders such as type 1 diabetes, hypothyroidism and Addison's disease (see Section 2.7, p. 115).

Table 36 Differential diagnosis of oligomenorrhoea/amenorrhoea according to gonadotrophins and prolactin.

Hypogonadotrophism	Excessive weight loss, exercise or stress, pubertal delay, Kallmann's syndrome, pituitary disease/treatment
Normogonadotrophic	PCOS, CAH, anatomical defects
Hypergonadotrophism	Turner's syndrome, premature menopause
Hyperprolactinaemia	Prolactinoma, stalk disconnection

CAH, congenital adrenal hyperplasia; PCOS, polycystic ovarian syndrome.

 Baird DT. Amenorrhoea. *Lancet* 1997; 350: 275–279.
Forti G, Krausz C. Evaluation and treatment of the infertile couple. *J Clin Endocrinol Metab* 1998; 83: 4177–4188.
Kyei-Mensah A, Jacobs HS. The investigation of female infertility. *Clin Endocrinol* 1995; 43: 251–255.

2.4.2 POLYCYSTIC OVARIAN SYNDROME

Polycystic ovarian syndrome (PCOS) describes the association of ovarian hyperandrogenism with chronic anovulatory cycles in females with polycystic ovaries.

Aetiology/pathophysiology

Although the aetiology of PCOS is unclear, there is evidence to suggest that it is a complex disorder reflecting interplay between genetic susceptibility and environmental factors. It is now recognized that decreased peripheral insulin sensitivity with consequent hyperinsulinaemia are key features of the metabolic disorder that is typical of PCOS. In addition, retention of insulin sensitivity by the ovary has been suggested to contribute to ovarian thecal androgen production (in response to insulin and IGF-1).

The risk of developing type 2 diabetes is approximately six-fold higher in women with PCOS than in the general population, and they frequently exhibit a dyslipidaemia typical of the metabolic syndrome (see Section 1.17, p. 39).

Epidemiology

PCOS is estimated to affect approximately 5% of women of reproductive age.

Clinical presentation

The symptoms of PCOS usually date from menarche and develop gradually. The most common presentation is with features of hyperandrogenism (hirsutism/acne) and menstrual irregularity (oligomenorrhoea or amenorrhoea).

Physical signs

Obesity and hirsutism (but not virilization) are common findings. About 5% of women exhibit acanthosis nigricans, which is a sign of insulin resistance.

Investigations

The choice of investigations should be guided by the clinical presentation:

Luteinizing hormone and follicle-stimulating hormone

The LH : FSH ratio may be increased to >2 (reflecting anovulatory cycles and a lack of progesterone to inhibit LH release). However, gonadotrophins are normal in a significant number (30–50%) of women who meet the other diagnostic criteria for PCOS.

Testosterone

Testosterone is often slightly increased (although usually <5 nmol/L, thereby distinguishing from androgen-secreting tumours).

Prolactin

Ten to 20% of cases have mildly elevated prolactin levels.

Fasting glucose/oral glucose tolerance test/lipid profile

Check for evidence of impaired glucose tolerance/frank DM and the dyslipidaemia of the metabolic syndrome.

Provera® withdrawal bleed

PCOS is not an oestrogen deficient state and therefore a withdrawal bleed typically follows progesterone treatment.

Pelvic ultrasonography

A pelvic ultrasound scan (preferably trans-vaginal) may reveal the typical ovarian appearance of multiple follicles ('string of pearls') with increased stroma. However, note that the presence of polycystic ovaries does not in itself indicate that the women has PCOS (approximately 20% of all women have polycystic changes on ultrasound, although only one-third of these have PCOS).

Further investigations

Other tests may be considered to screen for:
- adult onset CAH (17–OHP)
- ovarian or adrenal tumours (DHEAS, androstenedione)
- Cushing's syndrome (see Section 2.1.1, p. 47).

Treatment

Weight loss

 There is good evidence to suggest that if patients manage to lose weight, this will ameliorate many of the features of PCOS.

Hirsutism/infertility

An approach to the management of hirsutism and infertility is outlined in Section 1.6, p. 15.

Metformin treatment

Several studies have suggested that metformin treatment

(e.g. 500 mg tds) in obese women with PCOS can regularize menses, reduce the frequency of anovulatory cycles and improve hirsutism. However, this is not yet a licensed use for metformin, and there remain questions about the optimum dose and safety in early pregnancy. Larger studies are awaited, both with metformin and other insulin sensitizers including the thiazolidinediones.

Other cardiovascular risks

In women with the metabolic form of PCOS, risk factors for coronary heart disease should be addressed, including type 2 diabetes, hypertension, hyperlipidaemia and smoking.

Prognosis

Epidemiological data has not confirmed the expected increase in the risk of coronary heart disease or cerebrovascular disease: some speculate that the excess risk conferred by insulin resistance is balanced by the protective effects of oestrogens.

Prevention

It has been suggested that if patients are targeted when they first present with mild hirsutism and oligomenorrhoea, and strongly encouraged to lose weight using whatever support systems are available, the progression of the syndrome to infertility can be avoided.

Franks S. Polycystic ovary syndrome. *N Engl J Med* 1995; 333: 853–861.

Hopkinson ZEC, Sattar N, Fleming R, Greer IA. Polycystic ovarian syndrome: the metabolic syndrome comes to gynaecology. *BMJ* 1998; 317: 329–332.

Wild S, Pierpoint T, McKeigue P, Jacobs H. Cardiovascular disease in women with polycystic ovary syndrome at long-term follow up: a retrospective cohort study. *Clin Endocrinol* 2000; 52: 595–600.

2.4.3 ERECTILE DYSFUNCTION

Aetiology and pathophysiology

Erectile dysfunction can be conveniently classified according to pathophysiology (Table 37).

Several different factors (e.g. diabetes, medication and anxiety) may contribute to the erectile dysfunction in any one patient. Furthermore, the psychological response to 'organic' impotence can be difficult to distinguish from primary psychogenic erectile dysfunction.

Table 37 Classification of erectile dysfunction.

Category	Examples
Psychogenic	Anxiety, depression, relationship problems
Drug-induced	β-Blockers, thiazides, many recreational drugs, alcohol
Neurogenic	Post-CVA, Parkinson's disease, spinal cord injury, pelvic surgery
Vascular	Hypertension, atherosclerosis, DM
Hormonal	Hypogonadism, hyperprolactinaemia
Chronic/systemic illness	Chronic renal failure, DM

CVA, cerebrovascular accident; DM, diabetes mellitus.

Epidemiology

General population

Impotence is estimated to affect 5% of men aged 40–50 years, 15% aged 50–60 years, 25% aged 60–70 years and 40% aged 70–80 years.

Men with diabetes

For men who were less than 30 years old when their diabetes was diagnosed, 45–50% will be impotent by 50 years of age and 60–70% will be impotent by 60 years of age.

Clinical presentation and physical signs

Erectile dysfunction should be distinguished from premature ejaculation or reduced libido. Penile curvature suggests Peyronie's disease. If the patient experiences masturbatory or early morning erections, this effectively excludes organic pathology and suggests a psychogenic basis.

Men may not volunteer the symptom of impotence. It is therefore important to ask 'at risk' groups, including those with diabetes, hypertension, atherosclerotic disease and hypopituitarism.

Investigation

The availability of the phosphodiesterase inhibitor sildenafil (Viagra®) has changed the investigation and management of erectile dysfunction.

Where applicable, a psychological evaluation should be arranged, and medication that could be causally related changed. It may then be appropriate to institute a therapeutic trial of sildenafil (see below) without further investigation, when the aetiology of the problem is clear (e.g. in a man with long-standing DM). Otherwise, a screen for systemic disease should be carried out, including full blood count, urea and electrolytes, glucose, cholesterol and PSA. Prolactin and testosterone levels should also be checked.

If the testosterone level is below the normal range, it

should be repeated in the morning, together with SHBG, LH and FSH concentrations.

- If the testosterone concentration remains low (less than 10 nmol/L) with an appropriately raised LH and FSH, a trial of androgen replacement therapy may be instituted
- If the pattern is that of hypogonadotrophic hypogonadism (low testosterone with low LH and FSH), assessment of anterior pituitary function together with imaging of the pituitary fossa is necessary (see Section 2.1.7, p. 57).

Treatment

Sildenafil (Viagra®)

Sildenafil selectively inhibits phosphodiesterase type 5, resulting in increased cyclic adenosine monophosphate (cAMP) concentrations in the glans penis, corpus cavernosum and corpus spongiosum, leading to increased smooth muscle relaxation and an improved erection. During clinical trials, 60% of attempts at intercourse were successful following Viagra® compared with 20% following placebo.

 Sildenafil augments the erectile response to sexual stimulation, but does not cause an erection to occur by itself. It is important that the patient understands that sexual activity must be attempted before the treatment is considered a failure.

Headache and flushing appear to be the most commonly experienced side effects. Contraindications to the use of sildenafil include nitrate therapy (risk of severe hypotension), significant cardiovascular disease and retinitis pigmentosa.

Urological treatment

Urologists may institute treatment with alprostadil (a synthetic form of prostaglandin E_1) either by intracavernosal injection or intraurethral application. Papaverine (a non-specific phosphodiesterase inhibitor) and phentolamine (α-adrenoceptor antagonist) may also be given by intracavernosal injection, often in combination or with alprostadil. Some men prefer the use of mechanical devices, such as vacuum constrictors. Various surgical treatments are available including penile prostheses and vascular procedures.

Androgen replacement

Where indicated, testosterone replacement should be instituted (see Section 2.1.7, p. 59).

Prognosis

Erectile dysfunction can have a considerable impact on a patient's quality of life, although one should not assume that all men (or all relationships) require sexual activity.

Prevention

Prevention of erectile dysfunction, particularly in patients with DM, includes optimal hypertensive and glycaemic control, appropriate treatment of lipids, not smoking and avoidance of excess alcohol.

 Levy A, Crowley T, Gingell C. *Clin Endocrinol* 2000; 52: 253–260.
Lue, TF. Erectile dysfunction. *N Engl J Med* 2000; 342(24): 1802–1813.
Morgentaler A. Male impotence. *Lancet* 1999; 354: 1713–1718.

2.4.4 GYNAECOMASTIA

Gynaecomastia denotes the presence of palpable breast tissue in a male.

Aetiology/pathophysiology

Gynaecomastia results from an increase in the net effective oestrogen : androgen ratio acting on the breast, either as a consequence of a decrease in androgen production/action, or an increase in oestrogen formation (including conversion of circulating androgens to oestrogens by aromatization). Physiological gynaecomastia may be seen in the newborn, at puberty and in the elderly. A significant number of cases are idiopathic. Other causes are listed in Table 38.

Epidemiology

Clinically apparent gynaecomastia is found at about 1% of autopsies, whilst histological changes have been reported in up to about 40%, suggesting that in many cases it may be a normal variant.

Clinical presentation

Significant points that should be noted include:
- age
- duration of enlargement
- local symptoms, e.g. tenderness, discharge
- drug history/alcohol use
- symptoms of thyroid disease or systemic illness.

Physical signs

It may be difficult to differentiate between gynaecomastia and 'lipomastia' (excess fat) in overweight subjects. Remember that a small number of cases of breast carcinoma arise in males—check for symmetry, discrete lumps and a nipple discharge. A full physical examination should be performed, noting in particular testicular size and symmetry (using an orchidometer—Fig. 8, p. 23), thyroid status and evidence of chronic liver disease.

Table 38 Causes of gynaecomastia.

Physiological	Neonatal
	Puberty
	Elderly
Idiopathic	—
Drugs that inhibit androgen synthesis or action*	Anti-androgens (e.g. cyproterone acetate, flutamide) or GnRH analogues, used in the treatment of prostate cancer
	Digoxin
	Spironolactone
	Ketoconazole, metronidazole
	Cimetidine
	'Recreational' use or abuse of anabolic steroids
Primary or secondary testosterone deficiency	Klinefelter's syndrome (XXY), Kallmann's syndrome
	Testicular failure secondary to mumps orchitis, trauma or orchidectomy
	Hyperprolactinaemia
	Renal failure
Increased oestrogen production (or increased aromatization)	Testicular, adrenal or bronchogenic tumours producing hCG, oestrogens or androgens
	Chronic liver disease
	Starvation
	Thyrotoxicosis

*Note that many other drugs have been implicated (some with no clear mechanism of action).
GnRH, gonadotrophin releasing hormone; hCG, human chorionic gonadotrophin.

Investigation

Some experts argue that gynaecomastia is so common that it should only be investigated when breast enlargement is symptomatic, progressive, has no simple explanation or is accompanied by abnormal findings on examination. In these circumstances laboratory assessment should include:

- renal, liver and TFTs
- LH, FSH and testosterone (±DHEAS)
- E_2 and hCG
- prolactin (if other clinical features of hyperprolactinaemia)
- karyotype analysis (especially if gynaecomastia is accompanied by tall stature and small testes suggestive of Klinefelter's syndrome).

If E_2 or hCG is elevated or testicular examination is abnormal, then a testicular ultrasound is indicated.

Treatment

Where identified, the underlying cause should be treated, including withdrawal, where possible, of any drug that is implicated. In idiopathic gynaecomastia, patients may simply need reassurance that there is no sinister underlying cause. Testosterone therapy is only effective in those cases associated with testicular failure. Tamoxifen may be of benefit in some patients. Cosmetic surgery is the only definitive treatment.

Complications

The principal problems associated with gynaecomastia are cosmetic and psychological. In young men, gynaecomastia may lead to teasing and social isolation. There is little evidence to suggest that gynaecomastia is associated with an excess risk of breast carcinoma, except in Kleinfelter's syndrome.

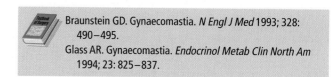

Braunstein GD. Gynaecomastia. *N Engl J Med* 1993; 328: 490–495.
Glass AR. Gynaecomastia. *Endocrinol Metab Clin North Am* 1994; 23: 825–837.

2.4.5 DELAYED GROWTH AND PUBERTY

Aetiology

Causes of pubertal delay and/or short stature are shown in Table 39.

Table 39 Aetiology of delayed growth and puberty.

Commonest causes of delayed growth and puberty	'Constitutional delay', a non-pathological condition, commoner in boys, which is often familial. Bone age is typically less than chronological age and the child usually achieves their predicted adult height
	Chronic/severe illness (e.g. coeliac disease, hypothyroidism, renal tubular acidosis, eating disorders and psychosocial deprivation)
Rarer causes of short stature	Chromosomal abnormalities (e.g. Down's syndrome, Turner's syndrome)
	Single-gene defects (e.g. the skeletal dysplasias such as achondroplasia)
	Dysmorphic syndromes (e.g. Prader–Willi syndrome)
	Endocrine disorders (e.g. growth hormone deficiency or resistance, pituitary disease and glucocorticoid excess)
Rarer causes of delayed puberty	Hypogonadotrophic hypogonadism (e.g. idiopathic, Kallmann's syndrome, pituitary dysfunction)
	Hypergonadotrophic hypogonadism (e.g. Turner's syndrome, Klinefelter's syndrome, gonadal dysgenesis, previous cytotoxic treatment or radiotherapy, trauma/orchitis in males, androgen insensitivity [testicular feminization])
	Androgen excess (e.g. CAH, adrenal or ovarian tumours)

CAH, congenital adrenal hyperplasia.

Clinical presentation and physical signs

Patients may present with short stature, failure to develop secondary sexual characteristics or primary amenorrhoea. It is important to determine whether there is a family history of delayed growth and puberty or a history of other childhood illnesses. Sections 1.8, p. 19 and 1.9, p. 22 outline the salient features that should be elicited from the history and physical examination.

Investigation

The average age of onset of puberty is $11\frac{1}{2}$ years in girls and 12 years in boys. In general, investigations should be initiated if there are no secondary sexual characteristics by 14 years in girls and $14\frac{1}{2}$ years in boys, and/or if the child's height falls below the 3rd centile and is inappropriate for the height of the parents. Remember, however, that up to 3% of children exhibit constitutional pubertal delay.

Routine blood tests/urinalysis

Initial evaluation should include screening for underlying disorders with:
- a full blood count
- urea and electrolytes (to check for chronic renal impairment)
- glucose
- CRP and/or ESR
- TFTs
- anti-gliadin antibodies (to exclude coeliac disease)
- plasma bicarbonate and urinalysis (to exclude renal tubular acidosis).

Gonadotrophins (luteinizing hormone and follicle-stimulating hormone) and oestradiol or testosterone

Whilst hypergonadotrphic hypogonadism suggests primary gonadal failure, hypogonadotrophic hypogonadism does not distinguish between constitutional delay (i.e. prepubertal levels) and secondary gonadal failure.

> **Bone age**
>
> Bone age (determined by radiograph) can be compared with chronological age to aid in the diagnosis of pubertal delay and allow predictions regarding potential future growth. For example:
> - low gonadotrophins and a more advanced bone age is suggestive of underlying pathology
> - low gonadotrophins and a relatively delayed bone age are more likely in the long term to be associated with normal pubertal development.

Karyotype analysis

The karyotype of all girls with delayed puberty and short stature should be checked, as the diagnosis of Turner's syndrome is not always clinically apparent (1 : 1500–1 : 2500 of live-born females—see Section 1.8, p. 19). Analysis may be necessary using DNA extracted from a second tissue (e.g. skin fibroblasts) in cases of mosaicism, where lymphocyte DNA is normal.

Similarly, males should be checked for possible Klinefelter's syndrome.

Further investigations

Depending on the results of these initial investigations, more complex tests of pituitary function (e.g. a GnRH test; assessment of GH status) may be indicated, together with structural studies, e.g. MRI of the pituitary fossa, visual field assessment and pelvic ultrasound.

Treatment

The choice of treatment will be directed by the underlying aetiology. Most children with constitutional delay of puberty, especially if mild, require only simple reassurance (they are normal, but their 'body clock' is starting later than that of their friends). Occasionally, psychological pressures are such that intervention may be indicated to 'start things off'. This typically involves the use of short-term low-dose sex steroids (<6 months), e.g. oestrogen treatment in girls (5–10 µg ethinyloestradiol per day) or testosterone injections (50–100 mg i.m. every 3–4 weeks) in boys. In both sexes, treatment is discontinued when the child's own pubertal development takes over.

Complications

The main problems associated with constitutional delay of growth and puberty are psychological and social. It is important to define the worries of the patient, their parents, and you (as their doctor): these may be different. Adolescence is a difficult time anyway, and short stature and sexual infantilism will exacerbate the usual problems. The child's behaviour may become immature or aggressive and antisocial. Parents may not allow the child the independence appropriate for their age, but may be inclined to 'baby' them. There may be bullying or teasing at school, with delays in developing social skills if they feel unable to start 'dating' at the same time as their peers. Contact with The Child Growth Foundation may be useful.

Buchanan CR. Abnormalities of growth and development in puberty. *J R Coll Physicians Lond* 2000; 34: 141–146.

Hindmarsh PC, Brook CGD. Short stature and growth hormone deficiency. *Clin Endocrinol* 1995; 43: 133–142.

Kulin HE. Delayed puberty. *J Clin Endocrinol Metab* 1996; 81: 3460–3464.

Stanhope R, Fry V. *Constitutional Delay of Growth and Puberty: A Guide for Parents and Patients.* The Child Growth Foundation, 1995.

2.5 Metabolic and bone diseases

2.5.1 HYPERLIPIDAEMIA

As with osteoporosis there is no easy definition of hyperlipidaemia. Instead attention focuses on how best to define those at high risk of developing coronary disease, based on the lipid profile and other risk factors.

Physiology/pathophysiology

Lipoproteins

The majority of lipids in plasma are contained within lipoproteins, which comprise a core of cholesterol, cholesterol esters and triglycerides, surrounded by a coat of proteins (principally apolipoproteins A, B, C and E) and phospholipids.

Lipoproteins can be divided into six major classes by ultracentrifugation or electrophoresis:

- chylomicrons (CM)
- very low density lipoproteins (VLDL)
- intermediate density lipoproteins (IDL)
- low density lipoproteins (LDL)
- high density lipoproteins (HDL)
- Lipoprotein(a) (Lp[a]).

Exogenous lipid pathway

CM are formed in the intestine from absorbed cholesterol and fatty acids and released into the circulation via the thoracic duct.

As they pass through the circulation, the majority of their triglyceride content is hydrolysed by the action of endothelial lipoprotein lipase in a process dependent on the presence of apoprotein (apo)-C-II.

The fatty acids released are taken up by skeletal muscle and adipose tissue and stored as re-esterified triglyceride or used as a source of energy.

The modified chylomicron remnants are taken up by the liver by a putative remnant receptor recognizing apo-E.

Thus the basic role of this exogenous lipid pathway is to deliver dietary cholesterol to the liver and fatty acids to the liver, skeletal muscle and adipose tissue.

Endogenous lipid pathway

VLDL are produced by the liver and form the starting point of the endogenous lipid pathway.

Like CM they are rich in triglycerides and are modified by lipoprotein lipase to form VLDL remnants and subsequently IDL.

IDL can be taken up by the liver and peripheral cells via the LDL receptor, or they can undergo further conversion to produce LDL.

The majority of LDL are removed by LDL-receptor mediated endocytosis in the liver, with a small amount taken up by peripheral cells such as monocytes/macrophages.

Low density lipoprotein metabolism

LDL-receptor mediated endocytosis is subject to negative feedback (i.e. as intracellular cholesterol increases LDL receptor expression diminishes).

By contrast, oxidatively modified LDL are taken up by scavenger receptors that exhibit no such feedback regulation. It is thought that this unregulated scavenger receptor mediated uptake of oxidized LDL contributes to the formation of the lipid-laden foam cells that are a characteristic feature of atherosclerotic plaques.

High density lipoprotein metabolism

Rather less is known about the metabolism of HDL. In general HDL tends to be antiatherogenic, removing cholesterol from peripheral tissues (reverse cholesterol transport) and acting as antioxidants.

Lipoprotein(a)

Lp(a) forms the final lipoprotein class, differing from LDL only by the additional presence of apo(a). Its physiological role is unknown.

Classification

The most accurate classification (the Fredrickson classification) defines hyperlipidaemia by the lipoprotein classes present in increased concentration. However, most laboratories do not perform ultracentrifugation or electrophoresis routinely, measuring instead total cholesterol, triglycerides and HDL cholesterol, with calculation of LDL cholesterol by the Friedewald formula. Hence, often only a working division into hypercholesterolaemia, hypertriglyceridaemia or mixed hyperlipidaemia is possible. However classified, all dyslipidaemias may be either primary (monogenic or polygenic) or secondary (Table 40).

Several of the monogenic hyperlipidaemias warrant brief mention:

- the molecular defect in familial hypercholesterolaemia involves the LDL receptor. In homozygotes there is minimal LDL uptake, with high (~ 20 mmol/L) levels of total and

Table 40 Classification of dyslipidaemia according to clinical phenotype, lipoprotein abnormality and Fredrickson class.

	Lp class	Fredrickson	Primary causes	Secondary causes
Hypercholesterolaemia	↑ LDL	IIa	Familial hypercholesterolaemia Polygenic hypercholesterolaemia	Hypothyroidism Obstructive jaundice Corticosteroids Anorexia nervosa
Hypertriglyceridaemia	↑ CM	I	Lipoprotein lipase deficiency Apo-CII deficiency	Diabetes Oral contraceptive pill
	↑ VLDL	IV	Familial combined hyperlipidaemia Familial hypertriglyceridaemia	Alcohol excess Thiazide diuretics
	↑ CM⁺ ↑ VLDL	V	Lipoprotein lipase deficiency Apo-CII deficiency	
Mixed dyslipidaemia	↑ Remnants	III	Familial dysbetalipoproteinaemia	Diabetes Obesity
	↑ VLDL⁺ ↑ LDL	IIb	Familial combined hyperlipidaemia	Nephrotic syndrome Renal failure Glycogen storage disease Paraproteinaemia

Apo, apoprotein; CM, chylomicrons; Lp, lipoproteins; LDL, low density lipoproteins; VLDL, very low density lipoproteins.

LDL cholesterol and a greatly increased risk of atherosclerosis. Heterozygotes have an intermediate phenotype
• type III hyperlipoproteinaemia is a classic example of gene–environment interaction; apo-E_2 homozygosity is required but in combination with some environmental factor (such as diabetes, obesity, hypothyroidism) to produce the characteristic lipid profile and clinical features.

Epidemiology

Several large-scale studies (e.g. multiple risk factor intervention trial (MRFIT), Framingham, prospective cardiovascular Münster study (PROCAM)) have examined the potential links between dyslipidaemia and IHD.

Epidemiological evidence suggests:
• an association between high levels of total and LDL cholesterol and risk of IHD
• the relationship between cholesterol and risk of IHD is curvilinear, a 10% increase in cholesterol conferring a 20% increase in risk
• an inverse relationship between HDL cholesterol and IHD risk
• a weak relationship between hypertriglyceridaemia and IHD risk, which has not been confirmed in all studies, although high triglycerides do seem to confer an increased risk in the presence of hypercholesterolaemia.

Clinical presentation

Hyperlipidaemia may present with IHD (myocardial infarction or angina) or other vascular disease. Alternatively, it may be uncovered in an asymptomatic patient screened because of a positive family history of premature IHD,

the presence of other risk factors for IHD, the existence of a known secondary cause of hyperlipidaemia, or because he/she exhibits the characteristic stigmata of one of these disorders (see below).

Relevant points in taking the history from a hyperlipidaemic patient include:
• past history of vascular disease
• assessment of lifestyle factors—diet, exercise, smoking, alcohol consumption
• family history of hyperlipidaemia, hypertension, premature IHD
• drug history
• past history or symptoms of diabetes, thyroid disease, liver or renal failure, myeloma.

Physical signs

Some of the stigmata of hyperlipidaemia (Fig. 40) are given in Table 41.

The examination of the hyperlipidaemic patient should include a search for evidence of vascular disease (e.g. carotid or femoral bruits, diminished peripheral pulses), features of other disorders associated with secondary hyperlipidaemia (e.g. DM, hypothyroidism, liver or renal failure) and an assessment of other risk factors (e.g. obesity or hypertension).

Investigation

Initial labororatory assessment should include a full blood count and ESR (± serum electrophoresis—to exclude myeloma), tests of renal, liver and thyroid function, fasting glucose and a baseline creatine kinase. A resting ECG may not be as useful as an exercise test. In all cases a full

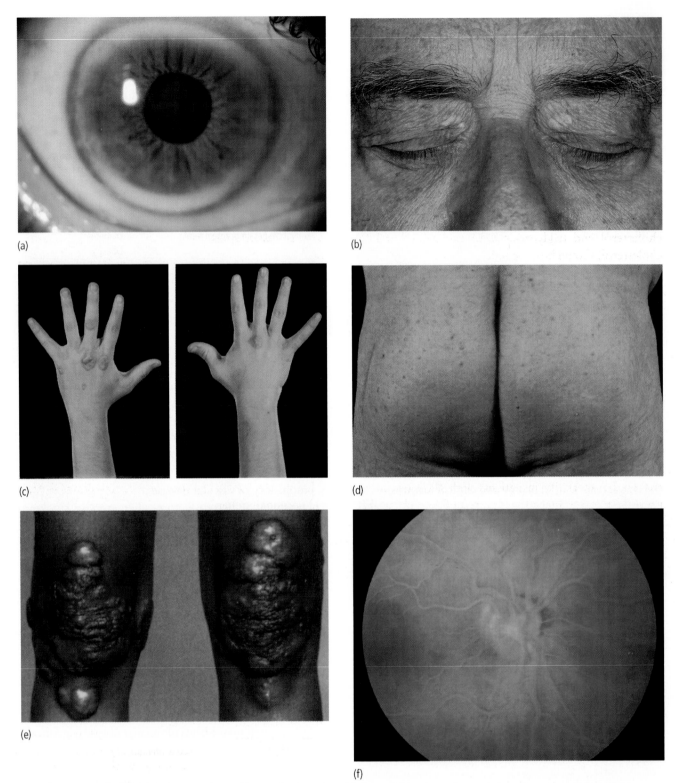

(a)

(b)

(c)

(d)

(e)

(f)

Fig. 40 Stigmata of hyperlipidaemia. Corneal arcus (a). Note the circumferential nature of this advanced arcus; in less advanced cases the upper eyelid may need to be retracted to expose the arcus. Xanthelasmata affecting both upper and lower eyelids (b). Tendon xanthomata over the extensor tendons of a patient with homozygous familial hypercholesterolaemia (c). Eruptive xanthomata. These appear classically over the buttocks, but can be more widespread (d). Tuberous xanthomata over the knees of a patient with mixed hyperlipidaemia (e). Lipaemia retinalis (f). Note the lipaemic appearance of all the retinal vessels, both arteries and veins.

Table 41 Stigmata of hyperlipidaemia.

↑ LDL–cholesterol	Corneal arcus
	Tendon xanthomata, e.g. of the Achilles' tendons
	Xanthelasmata
Mixed hyperlipidaemia	Tuberous xanthomata
	Eruptive xanthomata
	Lipaemia retinalis
Type III hyperlipidaemia	Linear xanthomata of the palmar creases

LDL, low density lipoproteins.

fasting lipid profile (with measurement of total and HDL cholesterol and triglycerides and calculation of LDL cholesterol) should be obtained.

Treatment

Given the high prevalence of IHD and the fact that many people who develop IHD appear to be at a relatively low risk, it is sensible to offer lifestyle advice to all (see Section 1.17, p. 39).

Secondary causes of hyperlipidaemia and other risk factors must be managed appropriately and subjects at high risk of IHD should be started on aspirin.

There is now abundant evidence that lipid-lowering drug therapy (with statins or fibrates) reduces IHD risk and overall mortality in patients with IHD (secondary prevention) or in subjects at high risk of developing IHD (primary prevention). Current recommendations are that patients with IHD and an LDL cholesterol >3.0 mmol/L after lifestyle modification should be treated with a statin. In primary prevention drug therapy should be considered in those in whom 10 years IHD risk exceeds 20%, and certainly offered to those in whom 10 years risk exceeds 30%. Convenient tables or computer programs for estimating 10-year risk based on age, sex, total : HDL cholesterol ratio, BP, diabetes and smoking status are now widely available.

Failure to achieve target (LDL cholesterol <3.0 mmol/L, HDL cholesterol >1.0 mmol/L and triglycerides <2.0 mmol/L) with monotherapy is an indication for referral to a lipid clinic.

 In general, statins should be given where the predominant problem is elevated LDL cholesterol and fibrates where there is significant hypertriglyceridaemia or low HDL cholesterol.

Complications

Both statins and fibrates are generally well tolerated, but patients should be monitored for the rare side effects of myalgia, raised creatine kinase and the development of abnormal liver function tests.

 Joint British recommendations on prevention of coronary heart disease in clinical practice. *Heart* 1998; 80(supplement 2): S1–S29.

2.5.2 PORPHYRIA

The porphyrias are a group of metabolic disorders resulting from defects in the enzymes of the haem synthetic pathway with consequent accumulation of various precursors. Clinically they may be divided into the acute and non-acute porphyrias (Table 42).

Pathophysiology

The haem synthetic pathway is shown in outline in Fig. 41.
• In both acute and non-acute porphyrias the reduced production of haem results in increased activity of δ-amino laevulinic acid (δ-ALA) synthetase as a consequence of impaired negative feedback
• In the acute porphyrias there is accumulation of δ-ALA and porphobilinogen
• In the non-acute porphyrias, however, increased porphobilinogen deaminase activity means there is no accumulation of δ-ALA or porphobilinogen.

The acute porphyrias are all dominantly inherited.

Clinical presentation

Acute porphyrias

Presentation is typically in early adult life with intermittent episodes characterized by:

Table 42 Classification of the porphyrias.

Acute porphyrias	Acute intermittent porphyria
	Variegate porphyria
	Hereditary coproporphyria
Non-acute porphyrias	Porphyria cutanea tarda
	Congenital porphyria
	Erythropoeitic, protoporphyria

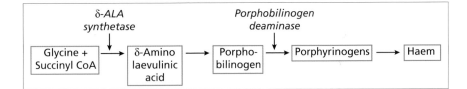

Fig. 41 Key steps in the haem synthetic pathway.

- acute abdominal pain and vomiting
- sensorimotor neuropathy, respiratory muscle weakness, coma, seizures
- psychiatric disturbance
- sinus tachycardia, hypertension and occasionally left ventricular failure.

Attacks may be precipitated by alcohol, sex steroids and a wide variety of drugs, especially barbiturates and other enzyme inducers. In variegate porphyria and hereditary coproporphyria (but not acute intermittent porphyria) these features are accompanied by the cutaneous features of porphyria cutanea tarda.

Non-acute porphyrias

The clinical features of each disorder include:
- porphyria cutanea tarda—a bullous photosensitive rash that heals by scarring; hepatomegaly; haemochromatosis
- congenital porphyria—a scarring bullous photosensitive rash; dystrophic nails; tooth discoloration; anaemia; splenomegaly
- protoporphyria—presentation in childhood; photosensitivity; peripheral paraesthesiae; hepatic dysfunction.

Investigation

During an attack of acute porphyria, porphyrin can usually be detected in fresh urine (red/brown on standing). Porphobilinogen in fresh urine can be detected by the development of a characteristic pink/red colour on mixing with Ehrlich's reagent, which is not absorbed out by butanol.

Treatment

Acute attacks are treated with supportive measures, a high carbohydrate intake and parenteral haem administration. β-Blockers, phenothiazines and benzodiazepines are safe treatments.

Following recovery, patients should be advised to abstain from alcohol, and given a list of drugs to be avoided (including oral contraceptives).
- Porphyria cutanea tarda is treated by venesection to reduce iron overload. Again alcohol should be avoided
- Congenital porphyria may be helped by low-dose chloroquine
- Protoporphyria can be helped by beta carotene and bile acid sequestrants.

See *Biochemistry and metabolism*, Section 6.
McColl KEL, Dover S, Fitzsimons E, Moore MR. Porphyrin metabolism and the porphyrias. In: *Oxford Textbook of Medicine*, 3rd edn, pp. 1388–1399. Oxford: Oxford University Press, 1996.

2.5.3 HAEMOCHROMATOSIS

Aetiology

The term haemochromatosis was introduced by von Recklinghausen in 1889 to describe the pathological accumulation of iron in a wide range of tissues producing organ dysfunction. It is most frequently due to a recessively inherited genetic disorder (adult, juvenile and neonatal forms), but may also complicate repeated blood transfusion, chronic iron ingestion and some forms of anaemia (thalassaemia, chronic haemolytic and dyserythropoietic anaemias).

Pathophysiology

Adult genetic haemochromatosis is usually due to mutations in the *HFE* gene on chromosome 6 (which is close to, and in linkage disequilibrium with, the gene for HLA-A3). Approximately 90% of cases are homozygous for the Cys282Tyr mutation (tyrosine replacing cysteine at residue 282). How this leads to pathological iron accumulation is uncertain, but it has been clearly shown that small intestinal iron absorption remains within normal limits, despite increased body iron stores in haemochromatosis.

Iron is involved in oxygen transport and redox reactions, but the mechanism of its cellular toxicity is not known. In haemochromatosis excess iron is found in almost all tissues, accompanied by cell loss and marked fibrosis, with the liver, pancreas, spleen, heart and other endocrine organs (anterior pituitary, testes and parathyroids) particularly affected. A similar pattern is seen in the other (secondary) causes of haemochromatosis.

Epidemiology

Genetic haemochromatosis is the commonest known inherited disease amongst Caucasians of north European descent, with a homozygote prevalence of between 0.1 and 0.5% (giving a gene frequency of 3–7%). Although the disease is present from birth, accumulation of iron and associated tissue damage take years to develop, with 70% of cases presenting between 40 and 70 years of age. Males are nine times as likely as females to develop disease, presumably reflecting menstrual loss that affords a degree of protection for women.

Clinical presentation

The classical triad of haemochromatosis comprises DM, hepatomegaly and slate grey skin pigmentation, but there are a wide range of symptoms related to:

Liver disease

• Cirrhosis—abdominal pain, fatigue, bruising.

Endocrine disease

• DM—polyuria, polydipsia, weight loss
• Hypogonadism—hair loss, diminished libido, impotence
• Hypoparathyroidism—weakness, tetany.

Cardiac disease

• Dilated cardiomyopathy—fatigue, breathlessness.

Arthritis

• Large joints with chondrocalcinosis
• Small joints resembling rheumatoid arthritis.

Arthritis occurs in about half of all cases, as does hypogonadism (usually hypogonadotrophic, but sometimes hypergonadotrophic), while cardiac disease occurs in approximately one-third.

Physical signs

The clinical signs of haemochromatosis include:
• slate grey skin pigmentation (82%)
• hepatomegaly (76%), with other stigmata of chronic liver disease
• testicular atrophy (50%)
• arthritis (46%)—especially second and third metacarpophalangeal joints and wrists
• splenomegaly (38%)
• cardiac disease (35%)—cardiomegaly, signs of biventricular failure
• diminished body hair (32%).

Investigation

Basic blood tests and radiology

Routine haematology and biochemistry should be sent, including liver function tests, clotting screen, and α-fetoprotein if hepatocellular carcinoma is suspected. Radiology may show deposition of calcium pyrophosphate (chondrocalcinosis) in large joints such as the knee.

Iron status

Demonstration of iron overload relies on an increased serum ferritin (in 70% of cases), increased serum iron, and plasma transferrin saturation greater than 62% (in 90% of cases).

Staining of liver biopsy specimens usually shows liver iron concentrations in excess of 1% (normally <0.15%). This used to be required for definitive diagnosis, but in at least some centres the need for liver biopsy has now been supplanted by genetic tests demonstrating homozygosity for the Cys282Tyr mutation of the *HFE* gene.

Treatment

Genetic haemochromatosis is best treated by venesection on a weekly basis until iron depletion is demonstrated by normalization of serum ferritin and transferrin saturation and the development of a mild anaemia. Thereafter, the frequency of venesection can be reduced to 1–2 monthly to prevent re-accumulation of iron stores.

Venesection has been shown to reduce the early mortality associated with untreated haemochromatosis, particularly cardiac or hepatic failure, but does not appear to reduce the risk of hepatocellular carcinoma or the severity of diabetes or arthritis. Given the efficacy of venesection, especially when instituted early in the course of the disease, identification of a case of haemochromatosis should be followed by screening of the relatives.

Diabetes, hypogonadism and hypoparathyroidism are managed according to standard guidelines.

Secondary haemochromatosis may be treated by parenteral administration of the chelating agent desferrioxamine.

Complications

Haemochromatosis carries an approximately three-fold increased risk of premature death due to hepatocellular carcinoma (32%), other malignancy (14%), cirrhosis (20%), DM (6%) or cardiomyopathy (6%). Patients must be kept under regular surveillance to allow treatment of arthritis and early detection of hepatocellular carcinoma.

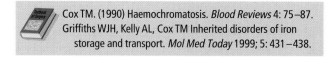

Cox TM. (1990) Haemochromatosis. *Blood Reviews* 4: 75–87. Griffiths WJH, Kelly AL, Cox TM Inherited disorders of iron storage and transport. *Mol Med Today* 1999; 5: 431–438.

2.5.4 OSTEOPOROSIS

Osteoporosis has been defined as 'a disease characterized by low bone mass and microarchitectural deterioration of the tissue, leading to enhanced bone fragility and a consequent increase in fracture risk'.

More pragmatic definitions of osteoporosis rely on measurement of bone mineral density (BMD), as it has been shown that a bone mass 1 SD below the mean peak bone mass of young adults carries a 1.5–2.5-fold increased risk of fracture. There is continuing debate as to whether the BMD should be compared with peak bone mass (the *t* score) or the age-adjusted bone mass (the *z* score). In fact,

Table 43 Secondary causes of osteoporosis.

Gastrointestinal disease	Coeliac disease, Crohn's disease, ulcerative colitits, gastrectomy, primary biliary cirrhosis
Endocrine disease	Cushing's syndrome, hyperparathyroidism, hypogonadism, hyperthyroidism, hypopituitarism, DM
Psychiatric disease	Anorexia nervosa, exercise-induced amenorrhoea
Others	Myeloma, mastocytosis, osteogenesis imperfecta, Gaucher's disease

DM, diabetes mellitus.

just as for hyperlipidaemia, the issue is not the definition of the disease but the identification of which patients should be treated.

Pathophysiology

Bone mass increases during growth and adolescence, peaks in the third decade and declines with age thereafter, with an increased rate of loss after the menopause in women. A number of factors influence bone mass including:
• genetic/racial—e.g. Afro-Caribbeans are much less likely to develop osteoporosis than Caucasians
• sex hormones—risk factors for osteoporosis include early menopause in women and hypogonadism in men
• environmental—inadequate calcium intake, physical inactivity, cigarette smoking and alcohol abuse.
• drugs—especially corticosteroids and long-term heparin.
In addition, osteoporosis may arise secondary to a large number of other medical conditions (Table 43).

 Bone mass is not the only determinant of fracture risk, which also depends on the quality and geometry of the bone, previous history of fracture and frequency of falls.

Epidemiology

It has been estimated that one-half of women and one-third of men in the UK will suffer an osteoporotic fracture in their lifetime. Twenty two and a half per cent of women and 5.8% of men aged over 50 in the UK have a BMD greater than 2.5 SD below the sex-adjusted mean peak BMD.

Clinical presentation

Osteoporosis typically presents with a low trauma fracture. Although any bone may be affected, the hip, vertebrae and distal forearms are classically involved. Relevant features to note in the history include:
• past medical history of major illness or any secondary cause of osteoporosis (including low BMI, i.e. <19 kg/m²)

• timing of puberty and menopause in females, history of prolonged oligo- or amenorrhoea
• average calcium intake
• exercise level
• current and previous drug treatment
• family history of osteoporotic fractures
• symptoms of gastrointestinal disease or malabsorption.

Physical signs

If left untreated, osteoporosis leads to progressive loss of height with increased kyphosis as a result of successive vertebral fractures.

Investigation

The principal objectives of investigation are to determine the overall risk of fracture and to identify any treatable cause of secondary osteoporosis.

Blood tests

 Osteoporosis is not a disorder of calcium metabolism, and therefore serum calcium, phosphate and alkaline phosphatase are usually normal.

Radiology

• Plain radiographs may demonstrate a fracture or vertebral collapse (Fig. 42)
• BMD, measured by dual energy X-ray absorptiometry (DEXA), is usually determined at the spine and hip (Fig. 43).

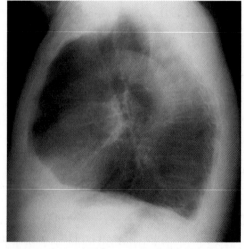

Fig. 42 Osteoporotic vertebral fractures. Lateral chest radiograph demonstrating loss of vertebral height and anterior wedging at several levels within the thoracic spine, leading to kyphosis. Preferential loss of trabecular over cortical bone gives rise to characteristic 'picture-frame' vertebrae.

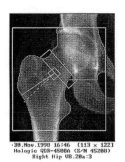
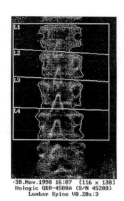

·30.Nov.1998 16:46 [113 x 122]
Hologic QDR-4500A (S/N 45200)
Right Hip V8.20a:3

·30.Nov.1998 16:07 [116 x 138]
Hologic QDR-4500A (S/N 45200)
Lumbar Spine V8.20a:3

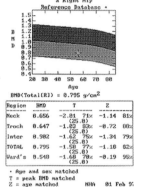
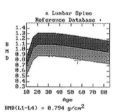

a Right Hip Reference Database ·

a Lumbar Spine Reference Database ·

BMD(Total(R)) = 0.795 g/cm²

Region	BMD	T	Z
Neck	0.656	-2.01 71% (25.0)	-1.14 81%
Troch	0.647	-1.03 93% (25.0)	-0.72 88%
Inter	0.982	-1.62 75% (25.0)	-1.34 79%
TOTAL	0.795	-1.58 77% (25.0)	-1.18 82%
Ward's	0.548	-1.60 70% (25.0)	-0.19 95%

· Age and sex matched
T = peak BMD matched
Z = age matched   NHA   01 Feb 97

BMD(L1-L4) = 0.794 g/cm²

Region	BMD	T(30.0)	Z
L1	0.702	-2.78 76%	-2.30 74%
L2	0.797	-2.70 73%	-2.18 77%
L3	0.830	-2.48 75%	-1.95 79%
L4	0.825	-2.91 72%	-2.37 76%
L1-L4	0.794	-2.70 73%	-2.19 77%

· Age and sex matched
T = peak BMD matched
Z = age matched   TK   04 Nov 91

Fig. 43 Bone densitometry. Dual energy X-ray absorptiometry (DEXA) bone mineral density scan in a man with osteoporosis secondary to long-standing hypogonadism. Values for the hip and lumbar spine are shown with both T and Z scores calculated for each site. The World Health Organization defines osteoporosis as a bone density >2.5 SD below the mean peak bone density in youth.

Treatment

Reduce fracture risk

The aim of treatment is to reduce the risk of fracture. Several agents are licensed for use in the UK, although not all have proven efficacy in terms of reducing vertebral and/or non-vertebral fractures.

Females

Treatment options include:
• exercise—regular exercise reduces fracture risk, but the magnitude of benefit is relatively small and requires a committed, maintained exercise regime
• calcium supplementation—decreases cortical bone loss and rates of fracture. Total calcium intake should be about 1500 mg per day, often requiring supplements of 500–1000 mg, combined with vitamin D (400–800 IU/day)
• HRT—in postmenopausal women HRT increases bone density and reduces fracture risk, but bone loss resumes once treatment is stopped
• selective oestrogen receptor modulators (SERMs), e.g. raloxifene—exhibit oestrogen-like agonist activity in some

tissues, e.g. bone, whilst acting as antioestrogens in others, e.g. breast
• bisphosphonates—increase BMD and decrease fracture risk, with a magnitude of benefit similar to HRT. They are particularly useful in steroid-induced bone loss. Etidronate at high dose can predispose to the development of osteomalacia, whilst alendronate can cause oesophageal ulcers, especially in those with gastro-oesophageal reflux disease. All the bisphosphonates have low bioavailability when taken orally and should be taken on an empty stomach
• vitamin D—although not a cause of true osteoporosis, vitamin D deficiency and osteomalacia may compound bone fragility in the elderly.

It is generally agreed that in women presenting with an osteoporotic fracture, first-line treatment lies between bisphosphonates, calcium supplements/vitamin D and HRT (or SERM). Postmenopausal females without fracture, but with low BMD, may be managed initially with HRT and calcium supplements/vitamin D, with the addition of bisphosphonates if serial bone density measurement shows no improvement.

Remember that combined oestrogen–progesterone preparations should be used in all females who have not undergone hysterectomy, to avoid the risk of developing endometrial hyperplasia and malignancy.

Males

Exercise, calcium/vitamin D supplementation and bisphosphonates are also central to the prevention and management of osteoporotic fractures in males. Testosterone replacement is reserved for hypogonadal cases.

Prophylaxis with steroid treatment

Patients who require prolonged treatment with high doses of steroids (equivalent to ≥7.5 mg of prednisolone per day) should receive calcium/vitamin D supplementation and be considered for treatment with a bisphosphonate for at least the duration of the steroid therapy.

Secondary osteoporosis

Where possible the underlying cause should be treated appropriately.

See *Rheumatology and clinical immunology*, Section 1.23.
Center J, Eisman J. The epidemiology and pathogenesis of osteoporosis. *Baillière's Clin Endocrinol Metab* 1997; 11: 23–62.
Reid IR. The management of osteoporosis. *Baillière's Clin Endocrinol Metab* 1997; 11: 63–81.

2.5.5 OSTEOMALACIA

Osteomalacia is the result of defective bone mineralization, leading to weakness and an increased propensity to fracture with subsequent deformity. If this occurs during childhood before fusion of the epiphyseal plates, it is known as rickets.

Pathophysiology

The formation of bone is a two-stage process involving the deposition of unmineralized matrix and its subsequent mineralization in a vitamin D dependent process, requiring normal osteoblast function. The metabolic pathways leading to the synthesis of the active form of vitamin D (1,25-dihydroxy-D$_3$) are shown in Fig. 44.

Table 44 lists the causes of osteomalacia; by far the commonest is reduced cutaneous production of vitamin D, which declines with age and is often exacerbated by reduced sunlight exposure and poor dietary intake. It is also more frequent following migration to a cooler climate, e.g. among Asian immigrants in the UK, where dietary consumption of phytates additionally impairs calcium absorption.

Epidemiology

Definitive diagnosis of osteomalacia depends on bone histology, so an accurate estimate of its prevalence is not possible. The biochemical features of osteomalacia are present in about 5% of the elderly population and up to 10–20% of patients with hip fractures.

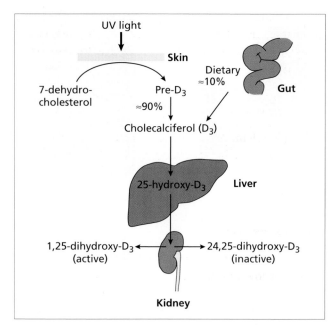

Fig. 44 Key steps in vitamin D metabolism.

Clinical presentation and physical signs

The presentation of osteomalacia is often vague and insidious with a gradual onset of generalized muscle aches and pains. A history of immigration, long-term anticonvulsant use, gastric surgery, coeliac disease or other malabsorption should prompt consideration of the diagnosis. Proximal myopathy may occur and manifest as difficulty rising out of a chair or in climbing stairs. Features of hypocalcaemia (see Section 2.5.9, p. 98) may be present. A significant proportion of patients presenting with a patho-

Table 44 Causes of osteomalacia.

Vitamin D deficiency	↓ Production	↓ Sunlight exposure
		↓ Dietary intake
		Malabsorption
		Liver disease
	↑ Clearance	Enzyme inducers, e.g. anticonvulsants
	↓ 1-Hydroxylation	Renal failure
		Vitamin D-dependent rickets type I (autosomal recessive)*
	↓ Action	Vitamin D-dependent rickets type II (autosomal recessive)†
Hypophosphataemia	↓ Intake	Antacids (phosphate binding)
	↑ Loss	Hypophosphataemic rickets (vitamin D resistant rickets—X-linked dominant)
		Fanconi syndrome
		Renal tubular acidosis
		Oncogenous osteomalacia
Defective mineralization		Hypophosphatasia
		High-dose etidronate
Defective bone matrix		Fibrogenesis imperfecta ossium

*Renal 25-hydroxy vitamin D 1α-hydroxylase deficiency.
†Absent or defective vitamin D receptor.

logical fracture have underlying osteomalacia. In childhood the characteristic features are of rickets with short stature, bowed legs and widened metaphyses (seen as 'rickety rosary' of the ribs).

Investigation

Although a definitive diagnosis of osteomalacia can only be made on bone biopsy, this is rarely indicated and most centres rely on biochemical and radiological evidence including:

Bone chemistry

- Low or low-normal serum calcium
- Low or low-normal serum phosphate (except in renal failure)
- Elevated serum alkaline phosphatase
- Vitamin D levels—if measured 1,25-dihydroxy-D_3 levels are often normal, albeit inappropriately so in the face of hypocalcaemia, hypophosphataemia and secondary hyperparathyroidism. Vitamin D-dependent rickets type II is an exception to the rule.

Many of the biochemical findings are attributable to progressive secondary hyperparathyroidism.

Radiographs

- Vertebrae—'cod-fish' appearance due to ballooning of intervertebral disc
- Pelvis, long bones, ribs—Looser's zones or 'pseudo-fractures', i.e. areas of low density representing unmineralized osteoid (Fig. 45)
- Rickets produces characteristic widening of the epiphyses with widening and cupping of the metaphyses.

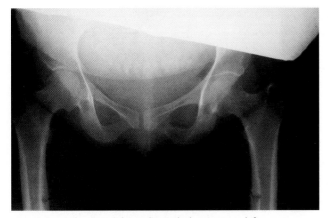

Fig. 45 Looser's zones. Pelvic radiograph showing pseudofractures (Looser's zones—areas of low density) in a patient with severe osteomalacia.

Treatment

Osteomalacia due to vitamin D deficiency is simply treated by dietary supplementation. The usual dose is 800–1000 IU per day. Calcium supplementation may also be required. The treatment of rickets secondary to phosphate wasting disorders requires oral supplementation sufficient to balance renal losses. Co-administration of vitamin D is often required to prevent hypocalcaemia. Any underlying disorder, e.g. coeliac disease should be managed appropriately.

Prognosis

With treatment hypocalcaemia, hypophosphataemia and any accompanying symptoms, including proximal myopathy, improve over several weeks. Alkaline phosphatase and PTH levels may take up to 6 months to normalize, during which time the bone remains weak and liable to fracture.

Francis RM, Selby PL. Osteomalacia. *Baillière's Clin Endocrinol Metab* 1997; 11: 145–163.

2.5.6 PAGET'S DISEASE

Paget's disease of bone was first described by Sir James Paget in 1879 as 'osteitis deformans'. It is characterized by grossly disordered bone formation giving rise to deformity and pain.

Pathophysiology

The primary disorder in Paget's disease appears to be an increase in the number and activity of osteoclasts, possibly secondary to viral infection. This is followed by increased osteoblastic activity, although the normal regulation of bone resorption and new bone formation is lost, with the production of hypertrophied, osteosclerotic bone. Bone deformity and pain are common, together with partial and pathological fractures. The disease process mainly affects the axial skeleton, skull and long bones, and frequently results in secondary osteoarthritis and nerve root entrapment.

Epidemiology

Approximately 3–4% of European and North American Caucasians aged 50 or over are affected. It is uncommon in other ethnic groups, including Asians.

Clinical presentation

Paget's disease is not infrequently an incidental radiological finding, or comes to light during the investigation of an elevated alkaline phosphatase noted on routine blood tests in an otherwise asymptomatic individual. Bone pain may reflect disease activity, which is often localized but multi-centric, although it can also arise as a result of partial or complete fractures. The deformed bone places abnormal stresses on adjacent joints with subsequent osteoarthritis. The characteristic bony deformities (bowing of long bones and thickening of the skull) may be noticed by the patient. Nerve root entrapment can affect any of the cranial nerves (classically the eighth nerve resulting in deafness), or spinal nerve roots. Occasionally enlargement of the base of the skull (platybasia) leads to paraplegia or acqueductal stenosis and hydrocephalus.

Physical signs

The characteristic physical signs reflect:

Bony deformities

- Enlargement of the skull with frontal bossing
- Bowing of long bones, especially the tibia
- Kyphosis of the skeleton.

Increased vascularity

- Warmth over affected bones
- Prominence of superficial temporal arteries
- High cardiac output (bounding pulse, cardiac failure).

Nerve entrapment

- Deafness.

Investigation

Biochemistry

- Alkaline phosphatase is usually raised, but without abnormalities of serum calcium or phosphate (except following prolonged immobility when hypercalcaemia may occur)
- An elevated 24-h urinary hydroxyproline excretion rate also indicates increased bone turnover.

Radiology

Plain radiographs

Plain radiographs may show localized enlargement of bone with cortical thickening and localized areas of both sclerosis and osteolysis (Fig. 46).

Radioisotope scanning

Radioisotope scanning with radiolabelled bisphosphonates allows demonstration of the full extent of bone involvement.

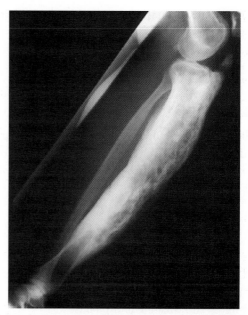

Fig. 46 Paget's disease of the tibia. Involvement of the weight-bearing long bones leads to bowing, particularly of the femur and, as shown here, the tibia ('sabre' tibia), which bow anteriorly and laterally. Note that the fibula is spared.

Treatment

The management of Paget's disease has been revolutionized by the bisphosphonates, which produce a prolonged, marked reduction of bone resorption by inhibiting osteoclast activity. Bisphosphonate administration is followed by decreased uptake on bone scanning, reduction in alkaline phosphatase, stabilization of hearing loss and improvement in other neurological dysfunction. Both pamidronate and alendronate are effective.

Accompanying arthritis requires suitable analgesia and knee or hip replacement as indicated.

Complications

In addition to the neurological (nerve entrapment), rheumatological (osteoarthritis), and cardiac (high-output cardiac failure) complications, osteosarcoma occurs in about 1% of cases; it is not yet known whether the risk is reduced by bisphosphonates.

 In a patient with Paget's disease, soft tissue swelling, increased pain or a rapidly rising alkaline phosphatase level should alert the clinician to the possibility of a developing osteosarcoma.

 Delmas PD, Meunier PJ. The management of Paget's disease of bone. *N Engl J Med* 1997; 336: 558–566.

2.5.7 PRIMARY HYPERPARATHYROIDISM

Pathophysiology

Primary hyperparathyroidism results from over-production of parathyroid hormone (PTH). There are normally four parathyroid glands, closely related to the thyroid, although occasionally there may be extra glands, e.g. ectopically sited in the superior mediastinum. Primary hyperparathyroidism is most frequently the result of a single adenoma, but in about 20% of cases there are multiple adenomata or diffuse hyperplasia of all four glands. Parathyroid carcinoma is rare (~1% of cases).

The excess PTH produces hypercalcaemia through three routes:
- increased osteoclastic bone resorption
- increased renal calcium reabsorption
- increased intestinal calcium absorption (mediated through increased vitamin D activity).

Epidemiology

The prevalence is estimated to be approximately 0.1–0.2%, affecting females twice as frequently as males.

Clinical presentation and physical signs

Asymptomatic hypercalcaemia, discovered on routine biochemical testing, is often the first indication of the diagnosis. A smaller number of cases present with hyperparathyroid renal disease (urolithiasis, nephrocalcinosis) or hyperparathyroid bone disease, leading to bone pain, especially once osteoporosis is established. Other features of hypercalcaemia may also be present (see Section 2.5.8, p. 97).

Investigation

Routine biochemistry

Hypercalcaemia is an almost universal finding in patients with primary hyperparathyroidism. The serum phosphate level is usually low-normal or low reflecting the effects of PTH in promoting urinary phosphate excretion. Alkaline phosphatase levels are typically normal or mildly elevated. Urea and electrolytes should be checked and occasionally more formal assessment of renal function, e.g. determination of glomerular filtration rate (GFR) is required. A 24 h collection for estimation of urinary calcium excretion should be performed to exclude familial hypocalciuric hypercalcaemia (FHH), an asymptomatic trait caused by loss-of-function mutations in the parathyroid calcium receptor.

Parathyroid hormone levels

Confirmation of the diagnosis can be made by determining the intact PTH level in a two-site assay (using monoclonal antibodies directed against both ends of the full-length PTH molecule), which fails to detect the smaller fragment PTH-related peptide (PTHrP). The finding of an elevated or normal PTH level is inappropriate in the setting of hypercalcaemia.

Radiology

Manifestations of hyperparathyroidism

The radiological hallmark of hyperparathyroid bone disease (osteitis fibrosa cystica) is the subperiosteal erosion, most easily seen in the distal phalanges of the fingers. A similar process in the skull results in the so-called 'pepper-pot' appearance. Occasionally osteolytic lesions are seen, suggesting the presence of bone cysts or 'brown tumours'. Long-standing hyperparathyroidism leads to generalized osteoporosis, which may be evident on plain radiographs. Nephrocalcinosis and urolithiasis are sometimes identified on plain abdominal radiographs or ultrasound examination of the renal tract (Fig. 47).

Localization of tumours

It has been argued by many that preoperative imaging is unnecessary, prior to initial surgical exploration in an uncomplicated case, and that an experienced surgeon should be able to determine the aetiology and effect the appropriate treatment for primary hyperparathyroidism. However, with the advent of minimally invasive parathyroid surgery (see below) and in cases of surgical re-exploration, localization studies including ultrasonography, [99m]technetium-sestamibi (Fig. 48), CT/MRI and/or venous sampling may be useful.

Treatment

Emergency/short-term

Hypercalcaemia should be treated as outlined in Section 2.5.8, p. 98.

Long-term

The definitive treatment of primary hyperparathyroidism is parathyroid gland surgery. Whilst it is widely accepted that virtually all symptomatic patients should be offered surgery, there is greater debate as to the appropriate management of apparently 'asymptomatic' individuals. For example, in one long-term follow up study neither

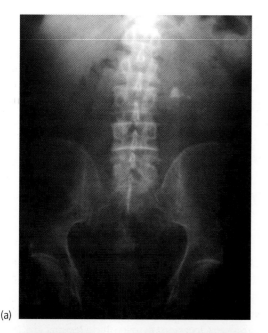

(a)

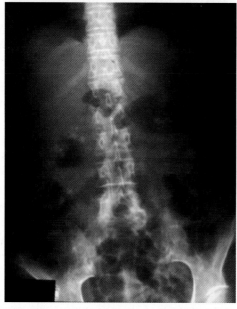

(b)

Fig. 47 Renal involvement in primary hyperparathyroidism. Plain abdominal radiographs demonstrating nephrolithiasis (a) and nephrocalcinosis (b) in the setting of primary hyperparathyroidism.

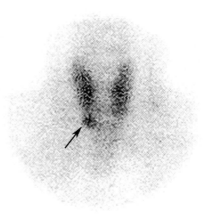

Fig. 48 Parathyroid adenoma. ^{99m}Technetium-sestamibi scan showing a parathyroid adenoma (arrow) in close proximity to the inferior pole of the right lobe of the thyroid gland.

When surgery is not undertaken, regular monitoring is required to check for disease progression/development of complications.

Some centres now offer minimally invasive parathyroid surgery, in which preoperative localization is used to guide the surgeon to the site of the adenoma, thus avoiding more formal neck exploration. Intra-operative PTH measurements help to confirm complete excision prior to closure, by virtue of the short half-life of PTH.

For the future, drugs are currently under trial that mimic the effect of calcium on the parathyroid calcium receptor and so decrease the synthesis and/or secretion of PTH.

Disease associations

Primary hyperparathyroidism occasionally occurs as part of the MEN syndromes (see Section 2.7, p. 115). In such cases there is usually four gland hyperplasia rather than a single adenoma.

Important information for patients

Where primary hyperparathyrodism is an incidental finding, the indications for and complications of surgery must be carefully discussed with the patient. The requirement for follow up, particularly if surgery is not initially undertaken, should also be stressed, and the patient advised to maintain adequate hydration (especially in hot weather) and to avoid thiazide diuretics.

 Utiger RD. Treatment of primary hyperparathyroidism. *N Engl J Med* 1999; 341: 1301–1302.
National Institute of Health. Consensus development conference 1991. Diagnosis and management of asymptomatic primary hyperparathyroidism. *Ann Intern Med* 1991; 114: 593.

the primary hyperparathyroidism nor its associated bone disease progressed over a 10-year period in the majority of cases. However, in approximately 25% significant worsening of osteoporosis was noted, as determined by serial bone densitometry. In addition, parathyroidectomy (when performed) corrected the abnormal biochemistry and produced a sustained increase in lumbar spine and femoral neck bone density in these 'asymptomatic' patients.

In general, parathyroid surgery should at least be offered to young patients (<50 years of age) and also to those with:
- symptomatic disease
- serum calcium >3 mmol/L
- radiological evidence of urolithiasis or nephrocalcinosis
- established osteoporosis.

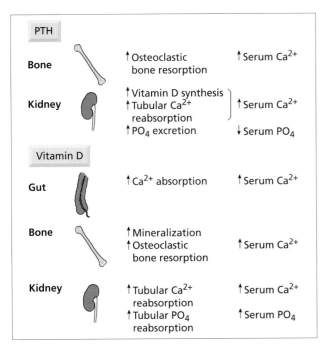

Fig. 49 Calcium homeostasis.

2.5.8 HYPERCALCAEMIA

Aetiology/pathophysiology

Regulation of calcium metabolism

The vast majority of body calcium is found in bone and teeth, with only about 1% in extracellular fluid and within cells. Of the extracellular calcium, approximately half is bound to protein (mainly albumin) or complexed to anions (phosphate, citrate and bicarbonate), with the other half existing as free ionized calcium (the bioavailable fraction). Hormonal control of extracellular calcium is exerted mainly by PTH and vitamin D (Fig. 49). Broadly speaking, the role of PTH is to act rapidly to maintain extracellular free calcium, whilst the actions of vitamin D are directed towards preserving skeletal calcium levels, both to act as structural support and as a reservoir of calcium.

Causes of hypercalcaemia

The major causes of hypercalcaemia are listed in Table 5, p. 8.

Hyperparathyroidism

Primary hyperparathyroidism is considered in Section 2.5.7, p. 95. Hyperparathyroidism can also arise in the context of abnormal calcium homeostasis in renal failure; in secondary hyperparathyroidism the response is appropriate and restores calcium levels to normal; however, in long-standing renal disease an autonomous inappropriate 'tertiary' hyperparathyroidism may arise with consequent hypercalcaemia.

Malignancy

Malignancy can lead to hypercalcaemia via a number of mechanisms including:
- osteolytic bone metastases (e.g. breast, bronchus, kidney or thyroid cancer)
- production of a PTHrP with PTH-like effects (e.g. squamous cell lung cancer)
- production of cytokines (e.g. osteoclast activating factor [OAF]) with bone resorbing activity, e.g. multiple myeloma
- production of vitamin D (e.g. lymphoma—rare).

Excess vitamin D activity

Increased production, or enhanced sensitivity to, vitamin D is thought to underlie the hypercalcaemia associated with sarcoidosis and tuberculosis, which is classically aggravated by exposure to sunlight. Vitamin D intoxication is an occasional cause of hypercalcaemia.

Clinical presentation and physical signs

Hypercalcaemia is often an incidental finding in an otherwise apparently asymptomatic individual. In others, symptoms and signs are varied and are perhaps best remembered according to the mnemonic 'stones, bones, abdominal groans and psychic moans':
- stones—renal colic (urolithiasis), polyuria and polydipsia (nephrogenic DI), nephrocalcinosis
- bones—arthritis and bone pain
- abdominal groans—nausea and vomiting, anorexia, constipation, peptic ulcer, pancreatitis
- psychic moans—lethargy, fatigue, depression, confusion, psychosis.

In addition, chronic hypercalcaemia may be associated with corneal calcification (band keratopathy). In all cases a thorough physical examination should be undertaken, looking for features which suggest an underlying cause, especially malignancy.

Investigation

Routine haematological and biochemical tests (full blood count, urea and electrolytes, liver function tests) should be performed on all patients presenting with hypercalcaemia, looking for evidence of malignancy (anaemia, abnormal liver chemistry) or renal impairment (suggesting possible tertiary hyperparathyroidism). Investigations that may specifically help to establish the underlying diagnosis, include:
- ESR—raised in malignancy, especially multiple myeloma
- phosphate—low in hyperparathyroidism, raised in multiple myeloma (particularly when accompanied by renal failure)
- alkaline phosphatase (bone isoenzyme)—reflecting osteoclast activation

• PTH—suppressed in virtually all causes of hypercalcaemia, except hyperparathyroidism where a detectable PTH level (normal or high) is inappropriate for the serum calcium level
• 24 h urinary calcium excretion—low in FHH (see Section 2.5.7, p. 95)
• chest radiograph—looking for primary or secondary malignancy, or hilar lymphadenopathy suggestive of sarcoidosis.

Other tests will be driven by the results of these initial investigations:
• serum electrophoresis, urinary testing for Bence-Jones proteinuria, and a skeletal survey if multiple myeloma is suspected
• isotope bone scan for bony metastases
• primary hyperparathyroidism—see Section 2.5.7, p. 95
• vitamin D levels may be helpful if intoxication is suspected, but require careful interpretation given their wide seasonal variation
• urinary catecholamines, thyroid function and synacthen tests as clinically indicated.

Treatment

Mild hypercalcaemia, detected as the result of routine biochemistry in an otherwise asymptomatic patient, may require no specific treatment. Such cases should, however, be investigated to establish the underlying cause.

Emergency/short-term

Reducing serum calcium levels

The following interventions are predominantly 'holding measures' that allow reduction in the serum calcium level whilst the underlying disorder is diagnosed and appropriate definitive treatment initiated.
• Re-hydration—hypercalcaemia is associated with nephrogenic DI, leading to polyuria and dehydration. Replenishment with normal saline (2–4 L per day depending on clinical status) is continued until the patient is fully rehydrated. A loop diuretic (e.g. furosemide [frusemide]) can be used to enhance the saline diuresis once the patient is no longer hypovolaemic
• Bisphosphonates—following initial rehydration, the drug of first choice for most patients is pamidronate. A dose of 30–90 mg, depending on the magnitude of hypercalcaemia, is administered by i.v. infusion over 4–6 h. Calcium levels typically fall over the next few days. The hypocalcaemic effect may persist for up to 6 weeks; further doses can be given
• Calcitonin (initially 5–10 IU/kg per day)—a useful alternative antiresorptive agent that is suitable for acutely lowering serum calcium levels in severe hypercalcaemia. Its beneficial effects are short lived, however, with most patients becoming refractory to treatment within a few day
• Glucocorticoids (e.g. prednisolone 40–60 mg per day)—limited use except in hypercalcaemia associated with haematological malignancy (e.g. multiple myeloma or lymphoma), sarcoidosis or vitamin D toxicity
• Mithramycin (plicamycin)—rarely used because of its toxicity (hepatic, renal, bone marrow).

Long-term

The long-term management of hypercalcaemia is directed at the underlying condition. Where such treatment fails to control hypercalcaemia, repeated therapy with bisphosphonates can be given. The need for adequate hydration, especially in hot weather, and avoidance of thiazide diuretics should be stressed in all cases.

Complications

Long-standing hypercalcaemia may result in ectopic calcification. Renal stones and nephrocalcinosis are both well described, as is widespread calcification of the medial layer of arterial walls. Hypercalcaemia is also a recognized cause of a shortened QT interval on the ECG.

Prognosis

In general, the prognosis is dictated by the underlying disease.

Bushinsky DA, Monk RD. Calcium. *N Engl J Med* 1998; 352: 306–311.

2.5.9 HYPOCALCAEMIA

Aetiology/pathophysiology

The causes of hypocalcaemia are listed in Table 45.

Since albumin is the principal calcium-binding protein in blood, hypoalbuminaemic states may be associated with apparent hypocalcaemia by virtue of reducing total calcium levels. Ionized calcium, however, remains unchanged. Accordingly, many laboratories routinely issue a 'corrected' calcium result, which includes an adjustment up or down from the measured level depending on whether the recorded albumin is below or above a defined 'normal' set-point, respectively.

The balance between total and ionized calcium is affected by acid–base balance and occasionally by the presence of anions such as citrate, such that a low ionized calcium, with the clinical features of hypocalcaemia, may occur in alkalosis and following extensive blood transfusion, even though the measured serum level lies within the normal range.

Hypoparathyroidism

In hypoparathyroidism PTH deficiency leads to:
• increased renal loss of calcium and retention of phosphate
• reduced bone resorption
• reduced calcium absorption (as a consequence of impaired 1-hydroxylation of 25-hydroxy vitamin D_3).
Serum phosphate levels are therefore high and alkaline phosphatase low.

Hypoparathyroidism most commonly arises in the setting of previous neck surgery, e.g. thyroidectomy. A period of

Table 45 Causes of hypocalcaemia.

Hypoparathyroidism	Post surgery
	Idiopathic/acquired
	Congenital
'Resistance' to action of PTH	Renal failure
	Drugs that impair osteoclastic bone resorption, e.g. bisphosphonates, calcitonin
	Pseudohypoparathyroidism
Vitamin D deficiency/resistance	
Acute pancreatitis	
Hypomagnaesaemia	Alcoholism
	Gastrointestinal losses
Hyperphosphataemia	Rhabdomyolysis
	Excessive phosphate administration
Malignant disease	

PTH, parathyroid hormone.

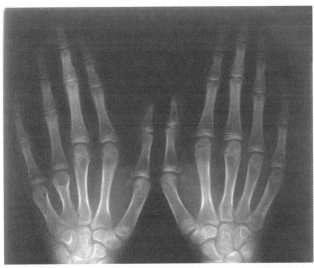

Fig. 50 Pseudohypoparathyroidism. Plain radiograph demonstrating the classical short 4th and 5th metacarpals of pseudohypoparathyroidism in the left hand compared with the normal appearances on the right.

transient hypocalcaemia may follow removal of a parathyroid adenoma, pending restoration of PTH secretion by the remaining intact glands. Occasionally this can be severe, reflecting avid uptake of calcium and phosphate by bone which has been chronically stimulated by PTH ('the hungry bone syndrome'). Idiopathic (acquired) hypoparathyroidism may occur as an isolated finding or is sometimes seen in the setting of the polyglandular endocrinopathies (see Section 2.7, p. 115).

Pseudohypoparathyroidism

Pseudohypoparathyroidism is a rare disorder resulting from target organ resistance to the action of PTH. The clinical and biochemical features of hypoparathyroidism are frequently accompanied by a characteristic somatic phenotype including short stature, a rounded face and short 4th and 5th metacarpals (Fig. 50). PTH levels are high. Interestingly, other family members may exhibit the somatic features without evidence of disordered calcium metabolism, so-called pseudopseudohypoparathyroidism.

Clinical presentation

Hypocalcaemia causes tetany, cramps, paraesthesiae of the extremities and muscle spasms precipitated by exercise or hypoxia. Seizure threshold is reduced and fits may occur. Chronic hypocalcaemia produces lethargy/malaise, and may mimic psychosis.

Physical signs

• In hypocalcaemia latent tetany can be provoked by inflating a sphygmomanometer cuff to 10–20 mmHg greater than systolic BP for 3 min. Carpopedal spasm results in the hand adopting a characteristic posture referred to as '*main d'accoucher*' (Trousseau's sign)

• Tapping the facial nerve in front of the ear may induce a brief contraction of the facial muscles on that side (Chvostek's sign).

Other manifestations of chronic hypocalcaemia include dystrophic nails, alopecia, subcapsular cataracts, papilloedema and occasionally movement disorders (reflecting basal ganglia calcification). Signs of other autoimmune endocrine failure (e.g. hypothyroidism, hypoadrenalism) may also be present.

Investigation

Relevant blood tests include urea and electrolytes (checking for renal failure), liver function tests (including albumin and alkaline phosphatase), serum calcium and phosphate. Arterial blood gases may be needed to confirm an underlying alkalosis. Further tests may include determination of $25(OH)D_3$ (the most reliable indicator of total body stores of vitamin D) and PTH levels, whilst a failure to increase urinary cAMP in response to infused PTH (the Ellsworth-Howard test) may be used to confirm resistance to PTH action in pseudohypoparathyroidism.

Treatment

Emergency

 In acute, severe symptomatic hypocalcaemia, i.v. calcium, given as 10 mL of 10% calcium gluconate (i.e. 90 mg of elemental calcium) over 5–10 min, should be followed by an infusion of 0.5–2.0 mg/kg per hour. Oral calcium and vitamin D should be commenced as soon as possible.

 If hypocalcaemia proves refractory to treatment, serum magnesium levels should also be checked.

Long-term

Specific underlying causes require appropriate management. As treatment with PTH is not available, hypoparathyroidism is managed using a combination of alfacalcidol (1α-hydroxycholecalciferol) or calcitriol (1,25(OH)$_2$D$_3$) together with calcium supplements (e.g. sandocal) as required. The dose must be carefully titrated, aiming to keep the serum calcium level in the low-normal range (thereby reducing the risk of nephrolithiasis and nephrocalcinosis).

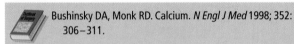 Bushinsky DA, Monk RD. Calcium. *N Engl J Med* 1998; 352: 306–311.

2.6 Diabetes mellitus

DM refers to a group of metabolic disorders characterized by hyperglycaemia, and resulting from inadequate production and/or impaired action of insulin. Table 46 outlines the current scheme for classification of this disorder.

Aetiology

See Table 47.

Table 46 Classification of diabetes mellitus (DM).

Type 1 (~20%)*	
Type 2 (~75%)†	
Specific types of diabetes (~5%)	Endocrine causes, e.g. Cushing's syndrome, acromegaly, phaeochromocytoma, glucagonoma
	Pancreatic causes, e.g. pancreatitis, trauma/neoplasia, pancreatectomy, haemochromatosis, cystic fibrosis
	Genetic causes, e.g. MODY (types 1–4), MELAS syndrome
	Drugs/chemical induced, e.g. glucocorticoids, thiazides, pentamidine
	Genetic syndromes associated with diabetes, e.g. Down's, Turner's, Klinefelter's, Lawrence–Moon–Biedel, Prader–Willi and dystrophia myotonica
Gestational diabetes	

*Type 1, previously called insulin dependent diabetes mellitus (IDDM).
†Type 2, previously called non-insulin dependent diabetes mellitus (NIDDM).
MELAS, myopathy, encephalopathy, lactic acidosis, strokes; MODY, maturity-onset diabetes of the young.

Type 1 diabetes

In genetically susceptible individuals, one or more environmental factors trigger immune-mediated destruction of islet β cells (insulinitis) leading to complete insulin deficiency.

Table 47 Aetiology and pathogenesis of diabetes mellitus (DM).

	Type 1	Type 2
Genetics	Polygenic. Several (>15) susceptibility loci have been identified (IDDM-1, IDDM-2, etc.). IDDM-1 is the major susceptibility locus, associated with *HLA* class II genes, situated on chromosome 6p. *HLA-DR3* and/or *DR4* are found in >90% of type 1 diabetics. *HLA-DQ* (a variant of *HLA-DQ* β gene) is more closely associated with diabetes. IDDM-2 is the insulin gene locus present on chromosome 11p and is also linked with diabetes	High identical twin concordance (60–100%), familial aggregation and varying prevalence in different ethnic populations suggest a strong genetic component. In only about 2% of cases has the genetic mutation been identified, e.g. MODY types 1 (*HNF 4α* gene), 2 (glucokinase gene) and 3 (*HNF 1α* gene); MELAS syndrome (mitochondrial DNA mutations)
Environmental factors	Viruses: coxsackie, rubella, mumps, CMV, EBV, etc. Dietary constituents: BSA in cow's milk, especially if infants are fed on it Nitrosamines in certain foods Stress	Strongly associated with obesity. BMI >35 kg/m^2 incurs a 40-fold increase in risk as compared to BMI <23 kg/m^2. Obesity is present in >two-thirds of type 2 patients and associated with insulin resistance. Malnutrition *in utero* may be linked with increased risk (fetal programming)
Aetiology	Evidence of autoimmunity: *HLA* genes on chromosome 6 are closely linked to immune modulation; association of type 1 diabetes with other autoimmune diseases; immunosuppressants can prolong β cell survival Mechanism of autoimmunity: probably T cell-mediated as there is a mononuclear cell infiltrate in the islets (insulinitis) Autoantibodies associated with type 1 diabetes: ICA are present in around 90% of newly diagnosed type 1 diabetics. Other antibodies present include GAD, tyrosine phosphate antibodies and IAA	Insulin resistance: whole body insulin resistance is present in type 2 diabetes. Increased secretion of insulin can limit hyperglycaemia but patients with coexisting β cell dysfunction are likely to develop diabetes Defects of insulin secretion: In type 2 diabetics insulin levels are low relative to the degree of hyperglycaemia, with blunting of the acute first phase and other abnormalities of stimulated insulin secretion. Diabetes results if insulin secretion can no longer compensate for the degree of insulin resistance present

BMI, body mass index; BSA, bovine serum albumin; CMV, cytomegalovirus; EBV, Epstein–Barr virus; GAD, glutamic acid decarboxylase; IAA, insulin auto-antibodies; ICA, islet cell antibodies; IDDM, insulin dependent diabetes mellitus; MELAS, myopathy, encephalopathy, lactic acidosis, strokes.

Type 2 diabetes

In the vast majority of type 2 diabetics the principal abnormality is one of reduced insulin sensitivity. In the very early phase of the disease euglycaemia may be maintained by increased insulin production. However, if insulin secretion is insufficient to compensate, impaired glucose tolerance or frank diabetes results. This typically occurs as a result of β cell exhaustion. Occasionally, insulin sensitivity is normal but insulin production is reduced (e.g. maturity-onset diabetes of the young [MODY]); diabetes again results.

Epidemiology

Type 1 diabetes

- Incidence increasing; high prevalence in Caucasians (Europe, North America and Australia)
- Typically young age at presentation. Peak incidence: 10–12 years of age.

Type 2 diabetes

- Prevalence increasing markedly, especially in developing countries; in the UK ~1–2% of Caucasians and up to 10% of Africans and Asians are affected
- Predominantly affects older people, with a peak incidence between 50 and 70 years of age.

Clinical presentation

The classic triad of diabetic symptoms consists of:
- polyuria
- increased thirst (polydipsia)
- weight loss.

These features (Table 48) typically manifest in an acute or subacute fashion in those with type 1 diabetes. By contrast, patients with type 2 diabetes often give a history of chronic progressive symptoms and it is not uncommon for complications to be present at the time of diagnosis or to form the presenting complaint. Unfortunately, some patients still present with acute decompensation of their previously unrecognized diabetic state:
- diabetic ketoacidosis (DKA) in type 1 diabetes
- hyperosmolar non-ketotic coma (HONK) in type 2 diabetes.

Physical signs

In younger type 1 diabetics there may be clinical evidence of weight loss, dehydration and ketosis. Older patients with type 2 diabetes not infrequently present with established complications. Those with secondary diabetes may

Table 48 Clinical features of diabetes mellitus (DM). Features of underlying conditions may be present in secondary diabetes.

Type 1	Type 2
Polyuria (++)	Polyuria (+)
Polydipsia (++)	Polydipsia (+)
Weight loss (+++)	Weight loss (+/−)
Tiredness (++)	Tiredness (+)
Blurred vision (+)	Blurred vision (+/−)
Balanitis, thrush, pruritis vulvae (+)	Balanitis, thrush, pruritis vulvae (++)
Neuritis (++)	Neuritis (+)
Presentation with DKA (not uncommon)	Presentation with HONK (rare)
Presentation with diabetic complications (rare)	Presentation with diabetic complications (common)

DKA, diabetic ketoacidosis; HONK, hyperosmolar non-ketotic coma.

have obvious features of the primary pathology, e.g. steroid excess, bronzing, acromegaly.

Drowsiness/coma, dehydration and hypotension are common findings in both DKA and HONK. Kussmaul respiration (indicating ketosis and acidosis) is usually limited to DKA. It is important to examine for evidence of a precipitating cause, e.g. infection or myocardial infarction.

Investigations

Urinalysis

Glycosuria may suggest the presence of diabetes but requires confirmation with a blood test. Conversely, absence of glycosuria does not exclude diabetes. The presence of ketones, blood, protein, nitrites and leucocytes should also be noted.

Blood glucose

The American Diabetes Association has recently recommended that the diagnosis of DM should be made on the basis of a fasting venous plasma glucose level of ≥7.0 mmol/L, which should be confirmed on a second occasion. It can also be made however, in a symptomatic patient whose random venous plasma glucose is ≥11.1 mmol/L (Table 49). There is currently on-going debate as to the role of the oral glucose tolerance test (OGTT) in routine practice.

Others

- Routine blood tests: urea and electrolytes, HbA_{1c}, lipid profile, thyroid function, liver chemistry
- ECG and chest radiograph (especially in the older patient)
- Retinal pictures/eye screening.

Table 49 Diagnosis of diabetes mellitus (DM). All values relate to venous blood.

Diagnosis	Fasting plasma glucose	Random plasma glucose
DM	≥7 mmol/L	≥11.1 mmol/L
Impaired fasting glucose	6.1–7 mmol/L	Not applicable

Treatment

Hyperglycaemic emergencies

Although the basic principles of management for DKA and HONK are similar, there are some important differences reflecting the distinction between absolute and relative insulin deficiency. For example:
• DKA occurs in type 1 diabetics lacking any insulin and is accompanied by ketosis and acidosis
• HONK arises in type 2 diabetics, with hyperosmolality the predominant biochemical feature.

Both may be precipitated by inadequate treatment (intentional, accidental or misguided) or physical stress such as infection, stroke or myocardial infarction.

 Remember that prompt treatment is required. Do not waste time performing unnecessary tests.

Urgent tests

In all cases check:
• laboratory glucose—to confirm hyperglycaemia
• urea and electrolytes—K^+ status; renal impairment
• full blood count—for neutrophilia (either as a feature of DKA or as a marker of infection)
• arterial blood gases/venous bicarbonate—for acidosis
• urinalysis—for ketones.

TESTS ACCORDING TO CLINICAL STATUS

Consider:
• CRP and a septic screen (blood cultures, chest radiograph and mid-stream urine)
• ECG and cardiac enzymes.

Urgent treatment

Both conditions carry a significant mortality (2–5% in DKA and up to 30% in HONK); treatment must be instituted promptly, beginning with basic supportive measures (to maintain airway, breathing and circulation).

FLUIDS

Dehydration and severe volume depletion (5–10 L) must be corrected as a matter of priority.

 • Aim to give 5–6 L within the first 24 h (e.g. 1 L over 1 h, followed by 1 L over 2 h, then 1 L over 4 h with 1 L every 4–8 h thereafter), but bear in mind the clinical setting, for example a fit 20-year-old is likely to tolerate more aggressive fluid replacement than an elderly patient with a history of cardiac disease. Consider central venous pressure (CVP) monitoring in the latter group
• Give an initial 500 mL bolus of colloid if hypotension (systolic BP <100 mmHg) is present, otherwise begin replacement with normal saline. Half normal saline is preferred if the serum sodium level exceeds 155 mmol/L; however, this must be accompanied by frequent (every 2 h) monitoring of the serum sodium to prevent a precipitous decline with consequent cerebral oedema. When the blood glucose falls below 12 mmol/L, 5% dextrose should be substituted in place of saline.

POTASSIUM

Acidosis often results in transient hyperkalaemia, and accordingly it is reasonable to omit potassium from the first bag of fluid whilst the results of electrolytes are awaited.

 Thereafter, beware of hypokalaemia, which may develop rapidly. Do not wait for the serum potassium to reach low levels before commencing replacement. Remember, insulin forces potassium inside cells and total body potassium levels are low. Electrolytes should be measured every 2 h in the initial stages and potassium added as required:
• serum (K^+) >5.0 mmol/L—none
• serum (K^+) 3.5–5.0 mmol/L—20 mmol KCl/L
• serum (K^+) <3.5 mmol/L—40 mmol KCl per L.

INSULIN

Add 50 U of soluble insulin to 49.5 mL of normal saline (1 U/mL) and infuse via a pump at a rate determined by the blood glucose level (Table 50), which should be checked every 1 h at the bedside. If there is any delay in obtaining a pump, give i.v. soluble insulin at a rate of 6 U per hour.

Table 50 Sliding scale for insulin infusion in diabetic ketoacidosis (DKA) and hyperosmolar non-ketotic coma (HONK). DKA may require higher infusion rates if the blood glucose level fails to fall during the first 1–2 h. By contrast, patients with HONK may require lower infusion rates to avoid dramatic falls in blood glucose with associated fluid shifts.

Blood glucose (mmol/L)	Insulin infusion rate (mL[U]/h)
<5	0.5
5.1–10.0	2.0
10.1–15.0	3.0
>15.0	6.0

OTHER CONSIDERATIONS

Consider:
• broad-spectrum intravenous antibiotics if there is any suspicion of an infectious precipitant
• insertion of a naso-gastric tube to prevent aspiration if the conscious level is depressed
• systemic anticoagulation in all cases of HONK, which is deemed to be a hypercoaguable state
• bicarbonate—but only in very sick patients with severe acidosis (pH <7.0). Give 200–500 mL of a 1.4% solution with additional KCl (20 mmol) over 30 min.

Transition to subcutaneous insulin/oral agents

Continue the insulin infusion until the patient is eating and drinking, and blood glucose is under control (<12 mmol/L) with no more than 1+ of ketonuria. In general, if in doubt it is safer to continue the infusion for a further 24 h to avoid the risk of 'rebound' hyperglycaemia. Transition to subcutaneous insulin should take place early in the day so that problems can be promptly dealt with. Give insulin s.c. 30 min before food and continue the i.v. infusion until the patient begins to eat.

Known type 1 diabetics can often be re-established on their original regimen (unless this contributed to the DKA), whilst newly diagnosed patients should be started on a 'gentle' b.d. regimen (see below). In some patients with HONK and no evidence of ketonuria, it may be possible to start on oral hypoglycaemic agents.

Ask the diabetes specialist nurse to see the patient prior to discharge and arrange follow up in a specialist clinic for appropriate education and advice.

Hypoglycaemia

Hypoglycaemia may occur in diabetics as a result of a missed or delayed meal, increased exercise, excess alcohol or following an overdose (usually non-deliberate) of insulin/sulphonylurea. The longer-acting, renally excreted sulphonylureas such as glibenclamide are particularly troublesome as they accumulate in patients with renal impairment and can cause severe, prolonged hypoglycaemia.

Clinical presentation

Apart from hunger, blurred vision and weakness, the major features of hypoglycaemia are either autonomic (e.g. sweating, tremor, palpitations) or neuroglycopaenic (e.g. headache, difficulty with concentration, drowsiness). The autonomic symptoms usually provide early warning of hypoglycaemia, but may disappear with autonomic neuropathy, adrenergic blocking drugs or recurrent hypoglycaemia. Occasionally, hypoglycaemia presents with seizures/hemiplegia.

Clinical presentation (continued)

• Mild episodes of hypoglycaemia are common and respond to simple measures, e.g. a sugary drink (to correct the hypoglycaemia) followed by a couple of biscuits or two slices of bread (to maintain euglycaemia)
• More severe hypoglycaemia may need assistance from others, e.g. application of a glucose gel (Hypostop) to the buccal mucosa or s.c./i.m. injection of glucagon (1 mg)
• If these measures fail, a bolus of i.v. glucose (e.g. 25 mL of 50% dextrose) should be given, followed if necessary by an infusion of 5 or 10% dextrose.

Re-educate the patient, with advice about alcohol, exercise and snacks. Nocturnal hypoglycaemia is much more likely if pre-bedtime glucose levels are <7 mmol/L. Determine whether there was an obvious precipitant and consider adjustments to the regular regimen.
Consider hospital admission:
• in the elderly or those who live alone
• when the cause is unclear or symptoms recur despite adequate treatment
• in the setting of sulphonylurea use or insulin overdose where hypoglycaemia may recur up to several hours later.

Short- and long-term management

Principal objectives

The principal objectives of the diabetes team are to:
• relieve symptoms and improve quality of life
• educate and empower the patient
• monitor control, adjust treatment and reduce other risk factors
• prevent and treat complications.

General approach

The management of diabetes requires a multidisciplinary team approach, involving doctors (physicians, GPs, orthopaedic and vascular surgeons, ophthalmologists and urologists), nurses (diabetes specialist nurses, practice and district nurses), dietitians, chiropodists and, most importantly of all, the patient.

A thorough history and examination should be carried out at the patient's first visit. Record details of presenting symptoms, past medical history (including hypertension and dyslipidaemia), family history and check for features suggestive of vascular disease. Ask about tobacco and alcohol use. Examine the cardiovascular (BP, peripheral pulses, etc.), and peripheral nervous systems, and assess the eyes, feet and skin. Where possible, arrange for the patient to see the diabetes specialist nurse and dietitian at the same visit, and consider referral for chiropody and retinal screening.

Glycaemic control

Several large prospective trials have shown that good glycaemic control reduces the risk of developing complications in diabetes (see below). Home monitoring (preferably finger-prick testing of blood glucose), together with periodic measurement of the HbA_{1c} (which reflects glycaemic control over the preceding 6–8 weeks), will indicate the level of diabetic control and the need for adjustment to therapy.

There are varying opinions as to what constitutes good or adequate glycaemic control. In general, blood glucose levels of 4–8 mmol/L are likely to correlate with a satisfactory HbA_{1c} (<7.0%). However, bear in mind the clinical setting: for example, whilst it is important to aim for tight control in a young type 1 diabetic, it may be necessary to accept more modest control in an elderly patient with type 2 diabetes who lives alone, and in whom it is important to avoid hypoglycaemia.

Landmark trials in diabetes

Diabetes Control and Complications Trial
Tight diabetic control with intensive insulin therapy (mean HbA_{1c} ~7%) reduced diabetic complications over a 7-year period in a cohort of type 1 diabetics. Risk of retinopathy was reduced by 60%, nephropathy by 30% and neuropathy by 20%. However, a two- to three-fold increased risk of severe hypoglycaemia was observed in the intensively treated group.

United Kingdom Prospective Diabetes Study
Good glycaemic control (median HbA_{1c} of 7% over a 10-year period) reduced the risk of microvascular complications in type 2 diabetics, whilst tight BP regulation decreased the risk of both microvascular and macrovascular complications. These benefits were, for the most part, independent of the agent used, although in obese patients metformin conferred particular advantage.

DIET AND LIFESTYLE MODIFICATIONS

Table 51 outlines key dietary and lifestyle issues for patients with diabetes.

INSULIN

Candidates for insulin
- All patients with type 1 diabetes
- Failed oral therapy in type 2 diabetes
- Type 2 diabetics during pregnancy (other than diet controlled)
- Type 2 diabetics during acute illness/surgery
- Patients with pancreatic failure/pancreatectomy.

Types of insulin
Table 52 describes the major classes of insulin currently in use.

Table 51 Diet and lifestyle advice for diabetics.

Category	Advice
Carbohydrates (50–55% of total calories)	Starchy carbohydrates with high fibre content, in which release occurs in a slow and uniform fashion
Fats (30–35% of total calories)	Polyunsaturates <10%, saturates <10% and monounsaturates >10% of the total
Proteins (10–20% of total calories)	If urinary albumin normal, 10–20% of total calories, if abnormal ≤10% of total calories†
Snacks*	Between meals and at bed time
Sugars	Avoid completely
Sweeteners	Aspartame and saccharin based are recommended
Diabetic food	Can be high in calories and expensive
BMI	Weight reduction: aim for BMI <25 kg/m²
Alcohol	Moderate consumption, especially of wine. Avoid excess beer
Exercise	Regular exercise is important to help reduce and maintain weight, to reduce insulin resistance and to improve BP and lipid control. It may increase the risk of hypoglycaemia
Smoking	Stop smoking

BMI, body mass index; BP, blood pressure.
* For those diabetic patients requiring insulin therapy.
† Some physicians consider protein restriction unnecessary.

Table 52 Types of insulin.*

Type	Action	Onset	Peak	Duration	Examples
Very rapid	Very rapid	15–30 min	1 h	5–6 h	Humalog®
Soluble	Short	30 min	1–2 h	6–8 h	Actrapid® Humulin S® Velosulin®
Isophane	Intermediate	2 h	4–6 h	8–12 h	Insulatard® Humulin I®
Zinc suspensions	Long	4 h	6–24 h	>24 h	Ultratard®

*Mixtures of soluble and isophane insulins (biphasic) are available, e.g. Mixtard® 10–50 and Humulin® M1–M5, containing 10–50% soluble insulin, respectively.

Which insulin?

Patients who are severely ill at diagnosis should be stabilized on an i.v. insulin infusion (see pp. 102–3). Less severely ill patients can be started on a twice-daily regimen, often most conveniently given as a biphasic (premixed) insulin. Subsequently, competent/motivated and younger patients are best managed with a 'basal-bolus' regimen with a night-time injection of an intermediate-acting insulin and three pre-meal injections of a short-acting insulin.

Occasionally, a continuous subcutaneous insulin infusion (CSII) is delivered via a small pump worn on a belt. However, this technique is expensive, associated with infection and weight gain and carries a risk of DKA due to technical failure or disconnection.

> • A phase of transient remission, referred to as the 'honeymoon period', frequently occurs shortly after starting treatment in patients with type 1 diabetes. Stopping insulin in this period is discouraged, as the need for insulin rapidly recurs
> • Whichever regimen is chosen, start cautiously and aim to avoid hypoglycaemia that would adversely affect the patient's confidence and make your job harder in the long run!

Side effects and complications

These may include:
• transient oedema and changes to lens refraction on starting insulin therapy
• lipohypertrophy (fatty lumps) at injection sites, especially if repeated in the same area (Fig. 51)
• lipoatrophy, although this is less common since the introduction of purified insulins (Fig. 51)
• hypoglycaemia.

ORAL THERAPY IN TYPE 2 DIABETES

An approach to the management of type 2 diabetes is outlined in Fig. 52. Most patients should undergo an initial 3-month trial of diet and lifestyle modification (Table 51), with tablets reserved for those who fail to achieve adequate control. Similarly, insulin can be used if diet and drugs fail to prevent hyperglycaemia.

Oral hypoglycaemic agents
See Table 53.

Follow up

The frequency of follow up will vary depending on the clinical context. However, even well-controlled patients should be reviewed every 6 months in a diabetic clinic (either at the local hospital or in the community with access to a Diabetic Centre) to aid early detection and treatment of complications. In addition to assessing glycaemic control, ask about symptoms of vascular disease (IHD,

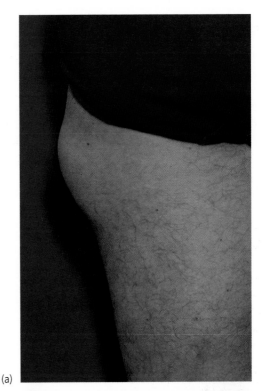

(a)

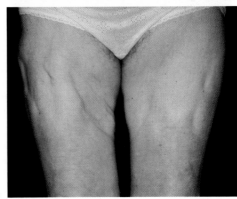

(b)

Fig. 51 Insulin-induced lipohypertrophy (a) and lipoatrophy (b).

cerebrovascular disease [CVD], peripheral vascular disease [PVD]), check for other macrovascular risk factors (especially smoking, hypertension, dyslipidaemia) and ask about features of neuropathy, including erectile dysfunction in males. Table 54 details those parameters which should be recorded at each visit.

Hypertension

It is now clear that aggressive BP control (≤140/80) is an essential part of the strategy to prevent micro- and macrovascular complications. If hypertension is detected, further investigations may be necessary to exclude secondary causes (see Section 1.18, p. 41). In those with evidence of nephropathy, there is evidence to suggest that the target BP should be even lower (≤130/80).

Although ACE-I are generally considered the antihypertensive agents of choice, especially in the presence of

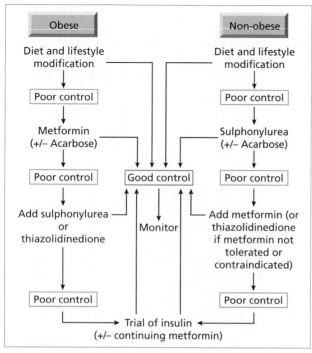

Fig. 52 An approach to the management of type 2 diabetes.

microalbuminuria/nephropathy, the United Kingdom Prospective Diabetes Study (UKPDS) demonstrated the β-blocker atenolol to be as efficacious as captopril in reducing micro- and macrovascular endpoints in type 2 diabetes, suggesting that it is the level of BP control which is the most important factor in determining outcome. Many patients require two or more agents to achieve their target BP. Calcium channel antagonists, α-blockers and diuretics are useful adjuncts, and angiotensin II antagonists may be tried in patients who are unable to tolerate ACE-I.

DYSLIPIDAEMIA

Clinical trials are in progress to define the exact role of lipid-lowering therapy in reducing the three-fold excess risk of macrovascular disease associated with diabetes. Post-hoc analysis of the recent statin trials suggests that diabetics appear to benefit at least as much as their non-diabetic counterparts from treatment with HMG-CoA reductase inhibitors.

Current guidelines suggest that, in the presence of vascular disease, diabetics should be treated to achieve an LDL

Table 53 Oral hypoglycaemic agents.

Agent	Examples	Action	Notes
Sulphonylureas	Gliclazide Glipizide Glibenclamide Glimepiride	Act (via the sulphonylurea receptor) to close β cell potassium channels, with subsequent calcium channel activation and insulin secretion	The drugs of choice in non-obese type 2 diabetics (reducing HbA_{1c} by up to 2%) In general, shorter-acting agents are preferred (e.g. gliclazide, glipizide) All can cause weight gain and hypoglycaemia
Biguanides	Metformin is the only biguanide currently licensed for use in the UK	Reduces hepatic glucose production and has beneficial effects on glucose uptake and metabolism (reducing HbA_{1c} by up to 2%)	Does not cause weight gain and is the treatment of choice in obese type 2 diabetics (reducing HbA_{1c} by up to 2%) It should be avoided in renal, liver and cardiac failure because of the risk of lactic acidosis. Side effects include nausea, vomiting, bloating, diarrhoea and a metallic taste Start with 500 mg once daily and gradually titrate upwards to minimize adverse effects
α-Glucosidase inhibitors	Acarbose	Blocks the breakdown of complex carbohydrates in the small intestine, thereby reducing the postprandial rise in blood glucose levels	Its use is limited by gastrointestinal side effects including flatulence, bloating, diarrhoea and abdominal cramps. It should therefore be started at low dose (50 mg/day) and gradually titrated upwards to a maximum of 100 mg tds. When combined with other oral hypoglycaemic agents, it produces a further small reduction in HbA_{1c} of ~0.5%. It does not induce weight gain. Liver function should be monitored during treatment
Thiazolidinediones	Rosiglitazone Pioglitazone	A novel class of antidiabetic agent that act as insulin sensitisers. High affinity ligands for a member of the nuclear receptor super-family-PPARγ	Currently licensed for use in the UK as add-on therapy with metformin in obese patients or with a sulphonylurea when metformin is contraindicated or not tolerated. In these circumstances, a further fall in HbA_{1c} of ~1% can be expected. Liver function should be checked prior to commencing treatment and monitored regularly thereafter
Prandial glucose regulators	Repaglinide	The first of a new generation of 'prandial glucose regulators' and acts via the sulphonylurea receptor	Principal advantage lies in its rapid onset of action allowing it to be taken with each meal

HbA_{1c}, glycosylated haemoglobin; PPARγ, peroxisome proliferator-activated receptor gamma.

Table 54 Diabetic follow-up: interim visits and annual review.

Check at each visit	Home monitoring record, HbA$_{1c}$, BMI, urinalysis, blood pressure. Continue education and assessment. Review and adjust treatment
Check once a year (i.e. annual review)	Clinical assessment: pulses, blood pressure, examine feet, visual acuity, fundi, injection sites
	Biochemical assessment: HbA$_{1c}$, urea and electrolytes, lipid profile, thyroid function, urinalysis, albumin : creatinine ratio (or other indicator of microalbuminuria)

BMI, body mass index; HbA$_{1c}$, glycosylated haemoglobin.

Table 55 Diabetic complications.

Macrovascular complications	Coronary artery disease Cerebrovascular disease Peripheral vascular disease
Microvascular complications	Diabetic eye disease Nephropathy Neuropathy
Specific complications	Diabetic feet Arthropathy and dermopathy Susceptibility to infections

cholesterol <3.0 mmol/L, an HDL cholesterol >1.0 mmol/L and fasting triglycerides <2.0 mmol/L. This also applies to any diabetic who does not have clinically apparent vascular disease, but whose annual risk (as calculated from available tables or computer programs) exceeds 3% (see Section 2.5.1, p. 87).

MICROALBUMINURIA

It is important to distinguish between:
- microalbuminuria—albumin excretion of 30–300 mg/24 h
- macroalbuminuria—albumin excretion of >300 mg/24 h ('stick positive')
- nephrotic syndrome—urinary protein loss of >3 g/24 h.

Microalbuminuria is a recognized risk factor for progression to full-blown diabetic nephropathy and macrovascular complications in both type 1 and type 2 diabetes. For example, 20–40% of type 1 diabetics with microalbuminuria will develop renal disease within 5 years. Although it is difficult to estimate its prevalence with certainty, approximately one-quarter of newly diagnosed type 2 diabetics have either micro- or macroalbuminuria.

All diabetics should be screened for evidence of microalbuminuria on an annual basis. Methods available include:
- semi-quantitative stick tests (e.g. Micral-Test® II)
- measurement of urinary albumin : creatinine ratio (positive if ≥2.0 in females and ≥3.0 in males)
- 24 h collection for urinary albumin excretion.

A positive result requires confirmation on a second occasion. A 24-h collection allows the extent of microalbuminuria/proteinuria to be determined. Once microalbuminuria has been diagnosed, it is important to achieve tight glycaemic control (HbA$_{1c}$ <7%) and to start treatment with an ACE-I, even in the absence of hypertension, which reduces the rate of progression to macroalbuminuria. Other risk factors for macrovascular complications must be rigorously controlled. The treatment of established diabetic nephropathy is dealt with below.

Complications

Diabetic complications (Table 55) are more likely with long-standing diabetes and with poor diabetic control.

Macrovascular complications

Diabetes is a major risk factor for the development of atherosclerosis and is associated with a much higher incidence of myocardial infarction, stroke and amputation. The presence of other risk factors such as smoking, hyperlipidaemia, hypertension and obesity compound the risk. Management follows the same principles as in non-diabetics, with rigorous control of other risk factors and appropriate use of antiplatelet agents, ACE inhibitors and β-blockers.

Microvascular complications

Diabetic eye disease

Retinopathy is the commonest microvascular complication (affecting almost all long-standing type 1 diabetics, and evident in ~20% of type 2 diabetics at presentation). The classification of diabetic eye disease is shown in Table 56.

Routine screening aims to detect eye disease before visual symptoms develop. Every diabetic must therefore undergo yearly examination including:
- visual acuity
- fundoscopy (through dilated pupils providing that there is no contraindication to tropicamide, e.g. glaucoma).

BACKGROUND RETINOPATHY

If background retinopathy is present (Table 56 and Fig. 53), fundoscopy should be repeated in 6 months. Review glycaemic control and treat associated hypertension. Check for evidence of microalbuminuria.

Microaneurysms and haemorrhages are more easily seen with the green lamp of the ophthalmoscope.

107

Table 56 Diabetic eye disease.

Retinopathy	Background	Microaneurysms
		Dot and blot haemorrhages
		Hard exudates
		Occasional (<5) cotton wool spots
	Pre-proliferative	Venous beading/looping
		Multiple haemorrhages
		Multiple cotton wool spots
		Intraretinal microvascular abnormalities
	Proliferative	Neovascularization around the disc
		Neovascularization elsewhere
Maculopathy		Oedema
		Hard exudates
Advanced diabetic eye disease		Retinal detachment
		Preretinal/vitreous haemorrhage
Cataract		

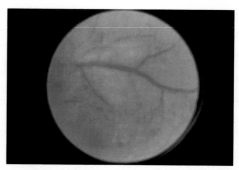

Fig. 54 Pre-proliferative diabetic retinopathy. Note the venous irregularity and beading.

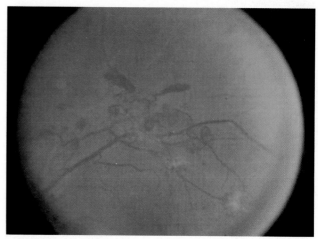

Fig. 55 Proliferative diabetic retinopathy. Note the leashes of new vessels and multiple haemorrhages.

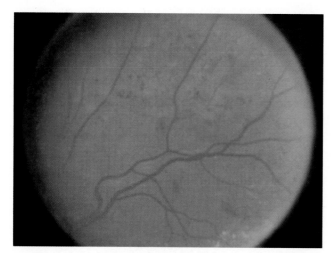

Fig. 53 Background diabetic retinopathy. Note the scattered red 'dots and blots' (microaneurysms and haemorrhages) and hard exudates (inferiorly).

PRE-PROLIFERATIVE RETINOPATHY

Multiple cotton wool spots indicate retinal ischaemia, and together with venous beading/looping and intraretinal microvascular abnormalities (IRMA) (intraretinal new vessels which, unlike 'classical' new vessels, do not lead to haemorrhage) constitute the changes of preproliferative retinopathy (Fig. 54). Prompt referral to an ophthalmologist is necessary for consideration for panretinal photocoagulation. Review glycaemic control and treat associated hypertension/microalbuminuria.

PROLIFERATIVE RETINOPATHY

If left unchecked, pre-proliferative changes may progress rapidly with the development of new retinal vessels, which are fragile and prone to haemorrhage, threatening vision (proliferative retinopathy—Fig. 55). Urgent referral to an ophthalmologist is necessary for laser treatment. Review glycaemic control; hypertension and microalbuminuria/nephropathy are likely to be present.

MACULOPATHY

Maculopathy is the commonest threat to vision in type 2 diabetics. It is often difficult to diagnose, although macular ischaemia should be suspected in the presence of circinate macular exudates ('macular star'—Fig. 56). Refer promptly to an ophthalmologist (for consideration for macular grid laser therapy). Again, address poor glycaemic control and hypertension.

ADVANCED DIABETIC EYE DISEASE

In advanced diabetic eye disease (Fig. 57) widespread neovascularization and haemorrhage may lead to traction retinal detachment, with preretinal or vitreous haemorrhage, presenting as sudden loss of vision.

CATARACTS

Cataracts are more common and occur at an earlier age in diabetics. They present with an insidious decline in visual

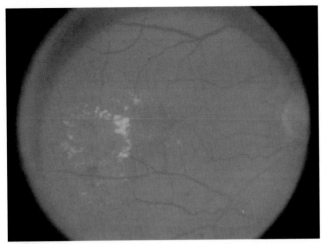

Fig. 56 Diabetic maculopathy. Note the ring of hard exudates encroaching on the macula.

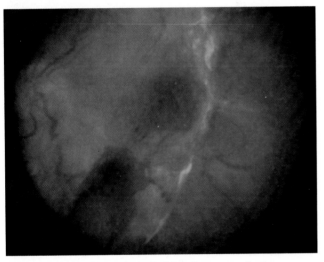

Fig. 57 Advanced retinopathy. Retinal detachment complicating extensive neovascularization and haemorrhage.

acuity. Occasionally 'snow-flake' cataracts may complicate acute hyperglycaemia, and these transiently worsen with imposition of good glycaemic control.

Nephropathy

Renal disease is a major cause of morbidity and premature mortality in the diabetic population. 'Nephropathy' is used to denote the presence of macroalbuminuria and a progressive decline in renal function (decreasing GFR and increasing serum creatinine), often accompanied by hypertension. Its incidence peaks when diabetes has been present for 15–20 years.

AETIOLOGY/PATHOGENESIS

It has been suggested that the elevated GFR seen at the onset of diabetes may predispose to the later development of renal disease, which is characterized by thickening of the glomerular basement membrane. Microalbuminuria (see above) is the earliest detectable change in the urine and progresses to intermittent and then persistent proteinuria. This is accompanied by mesangial expansion and then nodular sclerosis (Kimmelstiel–Wilson nodules). Eventually, glomeruli are replaced by hyaline material.

Although serum creatinine remains normal during the early stages, once persistent proteinuria develops it takes only 5–10 years to reach end-stage renal failure. Other causes of renal failure are present in 10% of type 1 and 30% of type 2 diabetics.

EPIDEMIOLOGY

Diabetic nephropathy develops in about 30% of type 1 diabetics, around 25% of Caucasian type 2 diabetics, but in up to 50% of type 2 diabetics of Asian and Afro-Caribbean origin, reflecting the earlier age of onset of diabetes and increased prevalence of hypertension in these groups. End-stage renal failure now occurs in fewer than 20% of type 1 diabetics, mainly because of aggressive treatment of hypertension.

CLINICAL PRESENTATION/PHYSICAL SIGNS

Nephropathy is usually detected during routine screening and patients are frequently asymptomatic at the time of presentation. When present, symptoms are those of uraemia (see *Nephrology*, Sections 1.5, 1.8 and 2.7.7).

Physical signs may include the pallor of anaemia, oedema from fluid overload, excoriations and associated features such as high BP or retinopathy.

INVESTIGATIONS

Diagnosis/initial assessment
Confirmation of a urinary albumin excretion of >300 mg/24 h indicates the presence of macroalbuminuria and should prompt a full assessment of renal function, including:
• serum electrolytes, urea and creatinine
• GFR or creatinine clearance (performed annually once nephropathy established)
• full blood count (for normocytic, normochromic anaemia)
• full lipid profile (for mixed dyslipidaemia).

Exclusion of other causes
Consider investigations to exclude other causes of proteinuria and renal impairment if there is little evidence of retinopathy to suggest microvascular disease elsewhere:
• midstream urine (for red cell casts and signs of infection)
• ESR, antinuclear factor, antineutrophil cytoplasmic antibodies (ANCA), anti-glomerular basement membrane (GBM) antibodies and complement levels
• calcium, urate, plasma and urinary protein electrophoresis

- renal tract ultrasound (to assess renal size and symmetry, and check for evidence of obstruction)
- magnetic resonance angiography (if renal artery stenosis suspected)
- renal biopsy (rarely required).

 Intravenous urography can precipitate acute renal failure, especially in the presence of dehydration or a serum creatinine >300 μmol/L.

TREATMENT

Established nephropathy

Once the urinary albumin excretion rate exceeds 300 mg per day, good BP control is the mainstay of treatment, using ACE inhibitors and other antihypertensives to keep BP <130/80. Diuretics may be needed for fluid overload and oedema. Drugs that are longer acting and predominantly renally excreted, e.g. glibenclamide, should be avoided. Metformin is contraindicated in renal failure (creatinine >150 μmol/L), due to the risk of lactic acidosis.

End-stage renal failure

Patients with nephropathy are best managed in a joint renal/diabetic clinic. Dialysis or renal transplantation is usually required at lower creatinine levels (around 500–550 μmol/L) than in non-diabetics. The preferred option is renal transplantation if co-morbidities permit.

PROGNOSIS

With effective renal replacement therapy, the main determinant of prognosis is now the associated vascular disease.

Diabetic neuropathy

Neuropathy is commoner in patients with a long history of diabetes, or those with poor glycaemic control.

 Classification of diabetic neuropathy

- Distal symmetrical (predominantly sensory) polyneuropathy
- Mononeuropathy and multiple mononeuropathy (peripheral or cranial nerve lesions)
- Diabetic amyotrophy (proximal motor neuropathy)
- Acute painful neuropathy
- Autonomic neuropathy.

DISTAL SYMMETRICAL POLYNEUROPATHY (PERIPHERAL NEUROPATHY)

This is the most common type of diabetic neuropathy and typically affects long peripheral nerves. There is loss of both myelinated and unmyelinated nerve fibres with segmental demyelination and axonal regeneration.

Clinical presentation

Pain (stabbing/burning/shooting), hyperaesthesia and hypo-aesthesia may be present, but up to 50% are asymptomatic.

Physical signs

Diminished or absent vibration sense and ankle jerks, together with an inability to feel the 10 g monofilament, are usually the earliest signs, and may be followed by diminished pain and temperature sensation. Muscular weakness and wasting are late features.

Investigations

Diagnosis is clinical, confirmed by nerve conduction and vibration perception threshold studies.

Treatment

The mainstay of treatment is good diabetic control. Tricyclic antidepressants (e.g. amitryptiline), anticonvulsants (e.g. carbamazepine or gabapentin) and topical capsaicin may help with symptom relief. Opsite (a semipermeable dressing) can provide local relief in hyperaesthetic areas.

Further complications

- Wasting of the small muscles of the hand
- High arched feet with clawing of toes
- Neuropathic ulcers leading to sepsis
- Neuropathic joints (Charcot's joints).

Prevention

Good glycaemic control reduces the risk of developing neuropathy. Patients should receive advice regarding foot care and undergo regular review by a chiropodist. Screening for peripheral neuropathy is essential as it is often asymptomatic.

MONONEUROPATHIES, DIABETIC AMYOTROPHY AND ACUTE PAINFUL NEUROPATHY

- Cranial mononeuropathies—typically affect the 3rd, 4th or 6th nerves. Pupillary responses are often spared in diabetic 3rd nerve palsy
- Radiculopathies—may involve any nerve roots, especially those affecting the trunk
- Diabetic amyotrophy (proximal motor neuropathy)—most commonly affects middle-aged men with long-standing type 2 diabetes, who present with asymmetrical painful wasting of the quadriceps muscles. It is often associated with anorexia and weight loss. Insulin is the mainstay of treatment even in those with apparent satisfactory glycaemic control. Symptoms gradually abate with time, although a significant number are left with residual disability

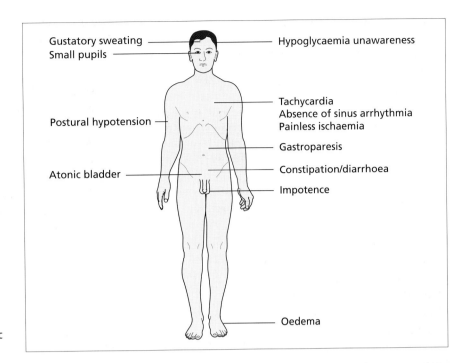

Fig. 58 Clinical features of diabetic autonomic neuropathy.

> • Acute painful neuropathy—pain (stabbing/burning/shooting) is usually severe and may be unremitting. Patients often report hyperaesthesia with marked tenderness of the skin to touch. Simple analgesia can be helpful, although opiates may be required. Tricyclic antidepressants (e.g. amitryptiline), anticonvulsants (e.g. carbamazepine or gabapentin) and topical capsaicin can be tried. Opsite may help in hyperaesthesia.

AUTONOMIC NEUROPATHY

Clinical presentation/physical signs
Autonomic neuropathy may manifest in a number of different ways (Fig. 58).

Investigations
Cardiovascular autonomic reflexes are most easily tested:
• lying and standing BP (a fall in systolic pressure >30 mmHg)
• absence of sinus arrhythmia (variation of <10 beats per min with deep breathing)

Erectile dysfunction should be investigated as outlined in Section 2.4.3, p. 80. Delayed gastric emptying can be documented with a radioisotope-labelled test meal.

Treatment
• Where possible, avoid drugs that cause postural hypotension. Treatment with fludrocortisone (50–100 µg per day) can be helpful in patients who are symptomatic
• Topical glycopyrrolate cream (0.5%) may be effective in gustatory sweating
• Consider metoclopramide (10 mg tds) or domperidone (10–20 mg tds) in those with upper gastrointestinal symptoms

• Codeine phosphate (30 mg qds) and other antidiarrhoeal agents provide symptom relief from diarrhoea. Tetracyclines are preferred for treatment of bacterial overgrowth
• The management of impotence is described in detail in Section 2.4.3, p. 81
• Intermittent self-catheterization (3–4 times a day) or placement of a long-term indwelling catheter is indicated for cases of neurogenic bladder.

Specific diabetic complications

The diabetic foot

Foot problems are very common and give rise to significant morbidity and mortality, accounting for the majority of hospital admissions in those with diabetes. Proper education and early detection can prevent many of the problems encountered. They are best considered in terms of the underlying pathology:
• neuropathic foot
• neuroischaemic foot
• neuropathic joints.

Table 57 outlines the major clinical features and approach to the investigation and management of the neuropathic and neuroischaemic foot.

NEUROPATHIC JOINT

Aetiology
The aetiology of neuropathic, or Charcot's, joints in diabetes is not fully understood. In the absence of pain, abnormal mechanical stresses may be borne recurrently across joint

Table 57 Clinical features, investigations and management of the diabetic foot.

	Neuropathic foot (Fig. 59)	Neuroischaemic foot (Fig. 60)
Presentation	Numbness, pain, calluses, ulcers, swelling	In addition to the features of neuropathy, patients may complain of intermittent claudication and/or rest pain
Physical signs	Evidence of sensory loss, absent ankle jerk, neuropathic oedema; calluses and ulcers at major pressure points, e.g. under the 1st and 5th metatarsal heads. Abscess and cellulitis. Charcot's joint. Good pulses	Cold foot with dependent rubor. Absence of pulses and trophic changes. Ulcers over the heel, dorsum of the foot and toes (often related to ill-fitting shoes). Gangrene or pre-gangrenous changes may be present
Investigations	Ulcer swab, blood cultures, blood glucose, blood count, biochemistry and urine for ketones. Radiograph of the foot/isotope bone scan (for osteomyelitis)	Doppler ultrasound to measure ABPI (normal >1.0; significant arterial occlusive disease is suggested by values <0.7). Arteriography may be indicated with a view to revascularization. Other investigations are as for neuropathic ulcer
Treatment	Remove callus, clean and debride. Antibiotics for infection. If osteomyelitis, cellulitis, abscess or sepsis present, arrange hospital admission for intravenous antibiotics and review of glycaemic control. Consider surgical/orthopaedic referral for drainage, debridement or amputation	Similar to the management of a neuropathic ulcer, but some patients may be suitable for angioplasty or a bypass graft, whilst others with critical ischaemia will require amputation
Complications	Trauma, infection, gangrene, amputation, Charcot's joint	Similar to those of the neuropathic foot, but with an increased risk of amputation if severe arterial disease is present

ABPI, ankle : brachial pressure index.

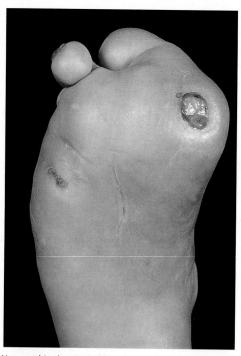

Fig. 59 Neuropathic ulcer. Typical 'punched-out' neuropathic ulcer in heavily callused skin underlying the 1st metatarsal head. Note the previous amputations.

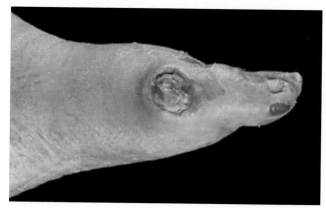

Fig. 60 Neuroischaemic foot. Classical ulceration reflecting both sensory neuropathy and vascular insufficiency.

surfaces. Surgery, even toe amputations, can change the normal weight-bearing axis and precipitate or accelerate the process.

Clinical presentation

Presentation is typically with a painful, 'hot' joint, especially the mid-foot. Discrimination from an infected joint can be difficult.

Investigation

Radiographs of the foot may be normal in the early stages but soon become abnormal with destruction and disorganization, particularly of the ankle and tarsometatarsal regions. An isotope bone scan may detect new bone formation and an MRI scan can be helpful, especially in differentiating from infection.

Treatment

Management involves bed rest initially and then mobilization with crutches or in a well-moulded total contact plaster cast until the swelling and warmth has settled. Improvement usually takes 2–3 months. Bisphosphonates (e.g. pamidronate 30–90 mg i.v.) may help to reduce bone resorption.

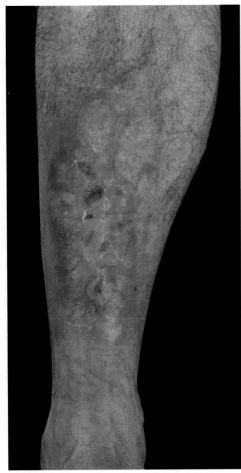

Fig. 61 Necrobiosis lipoidica diabeticorum.

Arthropathy and skin lesions

In addition to leg ulcers and fungal or bacterial infections of the skin, diabetics may develop:
• granuloma annulare—a cluster of small papules that typically form a ring on the back of hands or feet. Usually recovers spontaneously, but cryotherapy or steroid injections may be used
• necrobiosis lipoidica diabeticorum (Fig. 61)—a patch of erythematous skin with a central yellow area of atrophy that may ulcerate. The shin is the commonest affected site. The lesions are chronic and rarely resolve. Topical steroids or injection may be used but are not of proven benefit
• cheiroarthropathy—predominantly affecting the small joints of the hands with inability to flatten the palmar surfaces of the hands together due to collagen thickening.

Susceptibility to infections

Patients with diabetes have impaired neutrophil and lymphocyte function, impaired tissue repair processes and may have poor perfusion of the tissues due to vascular disease. There is a higher incidence of boils, abscesses, cellulitis

and fungal skin and mucosal infections (e.g. balanitis and thrush) amongst diabetics, who are also at risk of developing chest and urinary tract infections and osteomyelitis.

 In a patient with frequent or slow-healing infections, diabetes must be excluded.

Important information for patients

Sick day rules

Stress increases insulin resistance and hepatic glucose production. Accordingly, type 1 diabetics need more insulin, and type 2 diabetics may require short-term insulin, under conditions of severe or acute stress. Patients must be advised never to stop or even reduce their insulin. Indeed, in intercurrent illness the insulin requirement may increase by 10–20%. Meals may be substituted with frequent snacks and drinks, especially in the presence of anorexia or nausea. Frequent monitoring of blood glucose is necessary.

 Sick day rules for diabetic patients
• Never stop or even reduce your insulin; illness usually increases your insulin requirement
• Seek help if you are unwell, especially with vomiting or diarrhoea and if you cannot keep food or fluid down. If your blood sugar rises above 20 mmol/L or remains above 15 mmol/L for 24 h or if your urine test is positive for ketones, seek urgent medical help.

Surgery

Operations on insulin-treated diabetics should be planned for early morning. The preceding day patients should have their usual evening insulin. Omit the morning dose on the day of the operation and commence a sliding scale insulin infusion (50 U soluble insulin in 49.5 mL of normal saline infused at a rate determined by the blood glucose level—Table 50, p. 102) together with an i.v. fluid infusion, typically 1 L of 5% dextrose containing 20 mmol/L KCl every 8 h. After the operation, change to regular therapy once the patient is stable and taking food and fluids.

Patients with tablet-controlled type 2 diabetes undergoing surgery are also best managed by means of a sliding scale regime. Diet-controlled type 2 diabetes may be managed by an intravenous fluid infusion and careful monitoring of blood glucose if the planned operation is relatively minor.

Adolescence

Many physiological, behavioural and psychosocial factors

complicate the management of diabetes during adolescence. Ideally, patients should attend a specific clinic for adolescent diabetics, where they can experience mutual support away from the delays and obvious complications on view in the adult clinic. Patient-sensitive education and encouragement are vital. Long-term complications and emergencies should be explained in a realistic but non-threatening fashion. Contraceptive advice is essential.

Younger patients may benefit from diabetic camps where informal education is provided and practical techniques are taught.

Pregnancy and diabetes mellitus

Pregnancy should be planned to ensure that diabetic control remains tight from the time of conception. Patients taking oral agents should be switched to insulin, ideally a frequent injection regimen (three or four times a day). Insulin requirements increase during pregnancy, especially during the third trimester. Frequent home blood glucose monitoring is encouraged, with the aim of achieving a fasting glucose of between 4 and 6 mmol/L and a postprandial glucose <8 mmol/L. Patients should preferably attend a joint diabetic and obstetric clinic and have the support of midwives and diabetes specialist nurses throughout. Aim for a normal vaginal delivery where possible.

> Poor diabetic control at conception and in early pregnancy can lead to fetal malformations and later in pregnancy to excessive fetal growth, hydramnios, prematurity and the respiratory distress syndrome.

Diabetics with established nephropathy are advised against pregnancy, as the outcome is poor, especially if the serum creatinine level is more than 200 μmol/L.

Patients must be screened for retinopathy in each trimester. Those with retinopathy are seen once a month and referred to an ophthalmologist.

Diabetics who are hypertensive (with or without nephropathy) require special care as their BP control is likely to deteriorate.

During labour patients should be placed on a sliding scale insulin and dextrose infusion. Insulin requirements drop sharply after delivery, especially if breast-feeding.

Gestational diabetes

'Gestational diabetes' comprises gestational impaired glucose tolerance (GIGT) and gestational DM (GDM).

Indications for the OGTT (see Section 3.1.7, p. 121) in pregnancy include obesity or excessive weight gain, glycosuria in the first trimester, glycosuria on two occasions in the second trimester, previous gestational diabetes, a previous baby over 4 kg in birth weight, early macrosomia on ultrasound or a family history of diabetes.

Try diet alone in mild cases but if postprandial blood glucose levels are >8 mmol/L, treat with insulin throughout pregnancy and labour. The OGTT should be repeated 6–8 weeks after delivery. Fifty per cent of patients with GDM and GIGT will develop overt diabetes over the next 10–20 years.

Driving

- All diabetics, other than diet controlled, are required by law to inform the Driver and Vehicle Licensing Agency (DVLA). Diabetics who are otherwise fit and do not suffer from blackouts are allowed to hold an ordinary driving licence. Healthy diabetics on diet or tablets may hold a group 2 licence (for large goods vehicles and passenger carrying vehicles) if they meet the usual requirements. Insulin-treated diabetics are not now allowed to hold a group 2 licence.
- All insulin-treated diabetics must always carry a supply of sugar in their car. They should not drive if there is fear of hypoglycaemia. If there are warning symptoms while driving they should stop immediately, switch off the ignition and test their blood glucose.

Exercise

Regular exercise is helpful in reducing BP, weight and lipid levels, and increases insulin sensitivity. Regular exercise for 20–30 min, three to five times a week should be encouraged. Diabetics are advised to carry sugar with them when exercising and to take a snack or meal high in complex carbohydrates afterwards. Those who take regular exercise should also be able to reduce their pre-exercise insulin dose.

The Diabetes Control and Complications Trial Research Group. The effect of intensive treatment of diabetes on the development of microvascular complications of DM. *N Engl J Med* 1993; 329: 304–309.

Levy D. *Practical Diabetes*. London: Greenwich Medical Media, 1999.

The United Kingdom Prospective Diabetes Study Group. Effect of intensive blood glucose control with metformin on complications in overweight patients with type 2 diabetes (UKPDS 34). *Lancet* 1998; 352: 854–865.

The United Kingdom Prospective Diabetes Study Group. Intensive blood glucose control with sulphonylureas or insulin compared with conventional treatment and risk of complications in patients with type 2 diabetes (UKPDS 33). *Lancet* 1998; 352: 837–853.

The United Kingdom Prospective Diabetes Study Group. Tight blood pressure control and risk of macrovascular and microvascular complications in type 2 diabetics (UKPDS 38). *BMJ* 1998; 317: 703–713.

2.7 Other endocrine disorders

2.7.1 MULTIPLE ENDOCRINE NEOPLASIA

Three multiple endocrine neoplasia (MEN) syndromes are recognized, each characterized by endocrinopathies in which several glands undergo hyperplastic or neoplastic transformation and become hyperfunctional [1,2]. Table 58 outlines the key features of each syndrome.

Management

Although the individual components of the MEN syndromes are managed along standard guidelines, the patient with MEN presents a special challenge, for example it is clearly important to first exclude/treat a phaeochromocytoma prior to embarking on thyroid or parathyroid surgery.

Screening

Genetic testing now complements biochemical screening in the identification of affected members of MEN kindreds, since a relatively small number of mutations within the RET proto-oncogene appear to account for the majority of cases of MEN-2. Accordingly, genetic screening using the polymerase chain reaction permits the identification of affected individuals, thus obviating the need for serial biochemical screening tests in unaffected family members. Some centres advise that all identified affected individuals should undergo prophylactic thyroidectomy (preferably in childhood), since the penetrance of medullary thyroid carcinoma (MTC) is so high, and these tumours tend to be aggressive. Clearly there are important ethical and legal issues attached to screening in MEN.

2.7.2 AUTOIMMUNE POLYGLANDULAR ENDOCRINOPATHIES

Two major polyglandular syndromes have been described in which autoimmune-mediated dysfunction of two or more endocrine glands is frequently associated with other non-endocrine autoimmune disorders [3]. Table 59 describes the main features of each condition.

Table 59 Autoimmune polyglandular syndromes.

Type	Type I	Type II (Schmidt's syndrome)
Epidemiology	Rare, ?-autosomal recessive Childhood onset	Autosomal dominant or sporadic Young adults: females > males
HLA association	Unknown	DR3, DR4
Common endocrinopathies	Hypoparathyroidism Adrenal insufficiency	Adrenal insufficiency Hypo- or hyperthyroidism Type 1 DM
Less common endocrinopathies	Gonadal failure Hypo- or hyperthyroidism Type 1 DM	Gonadal failure
Non-endocrine manifestations	Mucocutaneous candidiasis Chronic active hepatitis Pernicious anaemia Vitiligo Alopecia	Myasthenia gravis Pernicious anaemia Vitiligo Alopecia

DM, diabetes mellitus.

Table 58 An overview of multiple endocrine neoplasia (MEN).

Type	MEN-1 (Wermer's syndrome)	MEN-2a (Sipple's syndrome)	MEN-2b (occasionally denoted as MEN-3)
Components	Parathyroid hyperplasia (≈80%) Pancreatic tumours (≈75%) Pituitary tumours (≈65%)	Medullary thyroid carcinoma (≈100%) Phaeochromocytoma (≈50%) Parathyroid hyperplasia (≈40%)	Mucosal neuromas (≈100%) Medullary thyroid carcinoma (≈90%) Marfanoid habitus (≈65%) Phaeochromocytoma (≈45%) (Parathyroid hyperplasia—rare)
Genetic locus	Chromosome 11 (The menin gene product is a tumour suppressor protein)	MEN-2a and MEN-2b are both associated with activating mutations in the RET proto-oncogene (α-receptor tyrosine kinase) on chromosome 10	
Clinical notes	Prolactinomas and non-functioning tumours are the most common pituitary lesions Gastrinomas (≈50%) and insulinomas (≈30%) form the bulk of pancreatic tumours	MTC (Note that MTC in the setting of MEN type 2b is particularly aggressive) Phaeochromocytoma Hyperparathyroidism is much more common in MEN-2a than MEN-2b Mucosal neuromas most commonly affect the oral cavity and gastrointestinal tract	

MEN-1, multiple endocrine neoplasia type 1; MEN-2a, multiple endocrine neoplasia type 2a; MEN-2b, multiple endocrine neoplasia type 2b; MEN-3, multiple endocrine neoplasia type 3; MTC, medullary thyroid carcinoma.

Hormone	Clinical syndrome	Tumours
ACTH	Cushing's syndrome	Oat cell bronchial carcinoma Thymoma Pancreatic carcinoma Bronchial carcinoid
ADH	SIADH	Oat cell bronchial carcinoma
PTHrP	Hypercalcaemia	Squamous cell bronchial carcinoma
OAF	Hypercalcaemia	Multiple myeloma Leukaemia
hCG	Clinical syndromes rare, but may include: Precocious puberty Gynaecomastia Menstrual irregularity	Testicular germ cell tumour Hepatocellular carcinoma Gastrointestinal tumour Choriocarcinoma
Erythropoietin	Polycythaemia	Renal cell carcinoma Cerebellar haemangioblastoma Uterine fibromas

Table 60 Ectopic hormone secretion by benign and malignant tumours and their associated clinical syndromes.

ACTH, adrenocorticotrophic hormone; ADH, antidiuretic hormone; hCG, human chorionic gonadotrophin; OAF, osteoclast activating factor; PTHrP, parathyroid hormone-related peptide; SIADH, syndrome of inappropriate antidiuretic hormone.

2.7.3 ECTOPIC HORMONE SYNDROMES

A number of tumours (benign and malignant) may be associated with ectopic hormone production and the development of a clinical syndrome due to hormone excess. Several examples are shown within Table 60.

1 Eng C. The RET proto-oncogene in multiple endocrine neoplasia type 2 and Hirchsprung's disease. *N Engl J Med* 1996; 335: 943–951.
2 Eng C, Ponder BAJ. Multiple endocrine neoplasia type 2 and medullary thyroid carcinoma. In: Grossman A (ed.). *Clinical Endocrinology*, 2nd edn, pp. 635–650. Oxford: Blackwell Science, 1998.
3 Asp A. Autoimmune polyglandular endocrinopathies. In: McDermott MT (ed.). *Endocrine Secrets*, 2nd edn, pp. 303–305. Philadelphia: Hanley and Belfus Inc, 1998.

3 Investigations and practical procedures

3.1 Stimulation tests

3.1.1 SHORT SYNACTHEN TEST

Principle

Administration of tetracosactrin (synthetic ACTH—'synACTHen') allows the acute adrenal response to ACTH to be assessed. In addition to promoting cortisol secretion, it also increases the production of other steroids in the biosynthetic pathway and can be used to exacerbate the enzyme block in differing types of CAH (see Section 2.2.4, p. 63), thereby confirming/excluding the diagnosis in patients with equivocal basal values.

Indications

- Diagnosis of both primary and secondary adrenal insufficiency
- Diagnosis of CAH.

Contraindications

Known allergy to synacthen. In addition, the manufacturers advise caution in subjects with asthma.

Practical details

Before investigation

In patients already on hydrocortisone replacement, the morning dose on the day of the test should be withheld until the test has been completed. Some centres also omit the evening dose on the day before the investigation.

The investigation

1 9.00 am. Take blood for serum cortisol and plasma ACTH; give synacthen 250 µg i.m. (or i.v.)
2 9.30 am. Take blood for serum cortisol
3 10.00 am. Take blood for serum cortisol
- ACTH samples should be taken on ice to the laboratory for immediate processing
- Low-dose synacthen (1 µg) is advocated by some as a more sensitive test of adrenocortical function
- For suspected CAH, measurement of 17-OHP is also required.

After investigation

Interpretation

ADRENAL INSUFFICIENCY

There is variation between laboratories as to the exact cut-off for a normal response. However, in general a serum cortisol level of >550 nmol/L at 30 min is taken to indicate an adequate adrenal reserve.

A subnormal response following synacthen suggests either:
- primary adrenal pathology
- secondary adrenal insufficiency (e.g. ACTH deficiency or exogenous steroid therapy) with consequent atrophy of the zonae fasciculata and reticularis.

The basal plasma ACTH level (providing it is taken properly and processed without delay) should help to distinguish between these two possibilities (high in primary adrenal failure). Alternatively, a long ('depot') synacthen test can be performed to confirm the persistent lack of responsiveness in primary adrenal failure, which contrasts with a delayed but detectable rise in cortisol in secondary adrenal insufficiency.

 A normal short synacthen test does not exclude partial pituitary ACTH deficiency (decreased pituitary reserve) in patients whose basal ACTH production is sufficient to prevent adrenal atrophy, but in whom the ACTH response to stress (e.g. insulin-induced hypoglycaemia) is attenuated.

CONGENITAL ADRENAL HYPERPLASIA

A peak 17-OHP level of >45 nmol/L confirms the diagnosis.

 Monson JP. How I investigate the hypothalamo–pituitary–adrenal axis and why. *CME Bulletin Endocrinology and Diabetes* 1999; 2(1): 12–15.

3.1.2 CORTICOTROPHIN-RELEASING HORMONE (CRH) TEST

Principle

Unlike pituitary corticotrophs, ectopic ACTH secreting tumours do not express CRH-receptors and are therefore not susceptible to stimulation by CRH. Accordingly, exogenous CRH administration can help to distinguish between pituitary-dependent Cushing's disease and ectopic ACTH secretion, either alone (see below) or in combination with inferior petrosal sinus sampling (see Section 2.1.1, p. 48).

Indications

To differentiate between Cushing's disease and ectopic ACTH secretion.

Contraindications

Known allergy to CRH.

Practical details

Before investigation

The patient should be fasted from midnight and warned that facial flushing is common following injection of CRH. Occasionally, transient hypotension occurs.

The investigation

1 Insert an i.v. cannula at 8.30 am with the patient recumbent. Take samples for measurement of serum cortisol and plasma ACTH 15 and 30 min later (−15 and 0 min samples)
2 Give synthetic CRH 100 μg i.v. at 9.00 am
3 Measure serum cortisol and plasma ACTH at 15, 30, 45, 60, 90 and 120 min.

After investigation

Interpretation

The majority of patients with Cushing's disease exhibit a normal or exaggerated increment in plasma ACTH and serum cortisol, contrasting with the lack of response from ectopic ACTH-secreting tumours.

Note, however, that up to 15% of pituitary adenomas may fail to respond to CRH.

Nieman LK, Oldfield EH, Wesley R *et al.* A simplified morning ovine corticotrophin-releasing hormone stimulation test for the differential diagnosis of ACTH-dependent Cushing's syndrome. *J Clin Endocrinol Metab* 1993; 77: 1308–1312.

3.1.3 THYROTROPHIN-RELEASING HORMONE TEST

Principle

Administration of thyrotrophin-releasing hormone (TRH) in normal subjects promotes release of pituitary TSH. This response is blunted in hyperthyroidism and exaggerated in primary hypothyroidism. An abnormal response may also be seen in hypothalamo–pituitary disorders. This test is rarely used now because of the availability of high precision TSH assays.

Indications

• Borderline cases of thyrotoxicosis (e.g. normal FT_4 and FT_3 with suppressed TSH)
• In the investigation of hypothalamo–pituitary disorders (e.g. as part of a combined pituitary triple test with insulin-induced hypoglycaemia and a GnRH test).

Contraindications

Known allergy to TRH.

Practical details

Before investigation

Non-fasting unless combined with an insulin tolerance test (see below). The patient should be warned that flushing and a desire to micturate are commonly experienced transient side effects.

The investigation

1 Insert i.v. cannula at 8.45 am (with the patient recumbent). Take blood for basal FT_4 and TSH levels immediately prior to TRH administration (0 min).
2 Give 200 μg of TRH i.v. at 9.00 am.
3 Take samples for TSH measurement at 20 and 60 min.

After investigation

Interpretation

• In normal controls TSH rises by at least 2 mU/L, with a 20 min value that is higher than the 60 min value
• In hyperthyroidism, the basal TSH level is suppressed and fails to respond to TRH
• Hypothyroidism due to hypothalamo–pituitary disorders may be associated with a subnormal or delayed TSH response.

Complications

Acute pituitary tumour haemorrhage/infarction has been reported following administration of TRH.

3.1.4 GONADOTROPHIN-RELEASING HORMONE TEST

Principle

Administration of gonadotrophin-releasing hormone (GnRH) in normal subjects leads to a prompt increase in serum LH, with a slower and lesser increment in serum FSH. This test is principally used to assess LH and FSH secretory reserves and does not *per se* diagnose gonado-trophin deficiency.

Indications

• As a part of a combined triple test in suspected hypopituitarism
• In the investigation of delayed puberty.

Contraindications

Known allergy to GnRH.

Practical details

Before investigation

Non-fasting unless combined with insulin tolerance test.

The investigation

1 Insert i.v. cannula at 8.45 am. Take samples for basal serum LH and FSH immediately prior to GnRH administration (0 min)
2 Give 100 μg of GnRH i.v. at 9.00 am
3 Obtain further samples for measurement of serum LH and FSH at 20 and 60 min.

After investigation

Interpretation

• In normal subjects, peak levels of LH are similar in both sexes (10–50 IU/L). Peak levels of FSH are generally lower (1–25 IU/L in females and 1–10 IU/L in males)
• In hypothalamo–pituitary disorders the GnRH response may be subnormal (especially in pituitary disease), normal or enhanced (particularly with hypothalamic dysfunction).

3.1.5 INSULIN TOLERANCE TEST

Principle

Insulin-induced hypoglycaemia is a powerful stimulus to cortisol and GH secretion.

Indications

The 'gold standard' test for the assessment of cortisol and GH reserves in patients with known or suspected hypothalamo–pituitary dysfunction.

Contraindications

• IHD, dysrhythmias and/or an abnormal resting ECG
• Epilepsy
• 9.00 am cortisol <100 nmol/L.

Practical details

Before the investigation

If there is any question of adrenal insufficiency, do not commence T_4 replacement to correct hypothyroidism until glucocorticoid replacement has been established—risk of precipitating a hypo-adrenal crisis. If in doubt, use an alternative, e.g. glucagon test.

• Check the resting ECG and ensure that 9.00 am serum cortisol is >100 nmol/L. Serum FT_4 should also be normal
• Liaise with the biochemistry laboratory in advance to ensure that glucose samples are assayed rapidly during the test and that the results are phoned through to you as soon as they are available
• 50 mL of 50% dextrose and 100 mg of hydrocortisone should be drawn up ready for use
• Nil by mouth from midnight
• Obtain the patient's consent, explaining the test and the symptoms of hypoglycaemia that they may experience (e.g. hunger, sweating, tachycardia, tremor). Reassure them that you will be present throughout
• Label the blood bottles
• Weigh the patient and calculate the dose of soluble insulin required: 0.15 U/kg (0.3 U/kg in those who are likely to be insulin resistant, e.g. Cushing's syndrome, acromegaly).

The investigation

1 Insert an i.v. cannula at 8.30 am
2 Take basal blood samples (for glucose, cortisol, ACTH and GH) at 9.00 am
3 Give the calculated dose of soluble insulin as an i.v. bolus
4 Take further blood samples at 20, 30, 45, 60, 90+/–120 min

5 Check a blood glucose test strip at each time point, but remember that this only provides an approximate guide to the degree of hypoglycaemia achieved

6 The blood glucose must fall to less than 2.2 mmol/L (laboratory sample) to provide an adequate stress

7 By 45 min you should expect the patient to experience symptoms of hypoglycaemia. If this does not occur and the blood sugar has not fallen below 2.2 mmol/L, you may need to administer another bolus of insulin and continue sampling for longer

8 Throughout the test you should record the patient's pulse and BP and note the presence or absence of symptoms of hypoglycaemia

9 Remember to reassure the patient as the test can be an unpleasant experience

10 If the patient becomes overwhelmingly hypoglycaemic during the test, administer 25 mL of 50% dextrose i.v. (repeated as necessary), and continue sampling, as the hypoglycaemic stimulus will have been sufficient. Consider giving hydrocortisone 100 mg i.v.

After the investigation

• Give oral glucose (e.g. Lucozade®) and lunch, and observe for 2 h
• Advise the patient to avoid exercise after the test (including cycling home!).

Interpretation

THE CORTISOL RESPONSE

A peak cortisol concentration of >580 nmol/L is generally accepted as a normal response, although some argue that a lower cut-off at 500 nmol/L is acceptable. In addition, an increment of at least 170 nmol/L from the basal level is expected.

THE GROWTH HORMONE RESPONSE

The definition of GH deficiency is controversial (see Section 2.1.7, p. 57). Most accept that a rise in GH to >20 mU/L denotes an acceptable response.

Complications

Provided the test is carried out according to these guidelines, it is associated with few serious adverse events.

Monson JP. How I investigate the hypothalamo–pituitary–adrenal axis and why. *CME Bulletin Endocrinology and Diabetes* 1999; 2(1): 12–15.
Orme SM, Peacey SR, Barth JH, Belchetz PE. Comparison of tests of stress-released cortisol secretion in pituitary disease. *Clin Endocrinol* 1996; 45: 135–40.

3.1.6 PENTAGASTRIN STIMULATION TEST

Principle

Although calcitonin is a useful marker for medullary thyroid carcinoma, levels may lie within the normal range in the early stages of tumour development or if C-cell hyperplasia (a premalignant stage) is present. Provocation with pentagastrin provides a sensitive method for detecting these early cases by inducing calcitonin release from the C-cells, with a correlation between the peak following the stimulus and C-cell mass.

Indications

To screen for medullary cell carcinoma in patients with MEN-2 or to identify at risk relatives.

Contraindications

Hypocalcaemia.

Practical details

Before investigation

• Check that both basal calcium and calcitonin levels are normal
• Restrict to a light diet with avoidance of alcohol for 12 h prior to the test
• Following pentagastrin, patients should be warned that they may experience several unpleasant side effects including flushing, nausea, chest tightness and abdominal cramps.

The investigation

1 With the patient supine, establish intravenous access. Take blood for measurement of basal plasma calcitonin
2 Give 0.5 µg/kg pentagastrin i.v. over 10–15 s
3 Repeat samples for calcitonin estimation at 2, 5 and 10 min.

 Blood should be transported immediately on ice to the laboratory for processing.

After investigation

Interpretation

An increment of two- to three-fold or greater following stimulation is usually taken as a positive result.

Important information for patients

It is of paramount importance that relatives understand the implications of this investigation as a screening test for medullary thyroid carcinoma and MEN-2.

 Eng C, Ponder BAJ. Multiple endocrine neoplasia type 2 and medullary thyroid carcinoma. In: Grossman A (ed.). *Clinical Endocrinolgy*, 2nd edn, pp. 635–650. Oxford: Blackwell Science, 1998.

3.1.7 ORAL GLUCOSE TOLERANCE TEST

Principle

Originally used to confirm/exclude the diagnosis of DM in individuals with equivocal fasting/random blood glucose levels.

Indications

Currently there is controversy over the role of the oral glucose tolerance test (OGTT) in routine practice (see Section 2.6, p. 100), although it is still used in pregnancy to diagnose impaired glucose tolerance and gestational DM (GDM).

Contraindications

None.

Practical details

Before investigation

Fast from midnight.

The investigation

1 Take a basal venous plasma glucose sample
2 Give 75 g of oral glucose (equivalent to approximately 390 mL of Lucozade®)
3 Take a further venous plasma glucose sample at 2 h.

After investigation

Interpretation

Values corresponding to a normal response, impaired glucose tolerance and frank DM are shown in Table 61.

Table 61 The oral glucose tolerance test in the diagnosis of diabetes mellitus (DM).

Diagnosis	Fasting glucose	2 h glucose
Normal	<6.1 mmol/L	<7.8 mmol/L
Impaired glucose tolerance	<7.0 mmol/L	≥7.8 but <11.1 mmol/L
Diabetes	≥7.0 mmol/L	≥11.1 mmol/L

3.2 Suppression tests

3.2.1 LOW-DOSE DEXAMETHASONE SUPPRESSION TEST

Principle

Unlike normal subjects, patients with Cushing's syndrome fail to fully suppress endogenous cortisol secretion following administration of dexamethasone.

Indications

Establishment of diagnosis of Cushing's syndrome.

Contraindications

• Severe intercurrent illness or infection
• Although not absolute contraindications, care should be taken in those with DM or active peptic ulcer disease.

Practical details

Before investigation

No specific preparation is required.

The investigation

1 **Day 0**. 9.00 am. Take blood for serum cortisol. A basal ACTH, if not already checked, can be measured on this sample
2 After venesection, give dexamethasone 0.5 mg orally every 6 h (i.e. at 9.00 am, 3.00 pm, 9.00 pm and 3.00 am) for 48 h
3 **Day 2**. 9.00 am. Take blood for serum cortisol (i.e. 6 h after last dose).

After investigation

Interpretation

In normal subjects, the basal serum cortisol lies within the reference range (200–700 nmol/L), but suppresses fully to undetectable levels (<50 nmol/L) following 48 h of dexamethasone, which does not cross-react in the cortisol assay.

Complications

Although the procedure itself has few complications, numerous circumstances can complicate interpretation of the results, with an apparent failure to fully suppress serum cortisol including:
- lack of compliance with dexamethasone (erroneous timing and/or missed doses)
- pseudo-Cushing's syndrome (see Section 2.1.1, p. 48)
- hepatic enzyme-inducing drugs (e.g. rifampicin, phenytoin may facilitate rapid metabolism of dexamethasone to levels such that there is failure to fully suppress a normal hypothalamo–pituitary–adrenal axis)
- cyclical Cushing's syndrome (see Section 2.1.1, p. 48) with normal dexamethasone suppression in the quiescent phase.

Important information for patients

If the test is being performed as an outpatient, it is important to provide the patient with clear instructions as to the timing of doses, and to check for any missed doses.

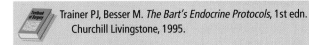
Trainer PJ, Besser M. *The Bart's Endocrine Protocols*, 1st edn. Churchill Livingstone, 1995.

3.2.2 HIGH-DOSE DEXAMETHASONE SUPPRESSION TEST

Principle

Unlike other causes of Cushing's syndrome, pituitary adenomas retain some sensitivity to glucocorticoid feedback such that ACTH release and consequently cortisol levels are reduced in response to high doses of exogenous steroid, e.g. dexamethasone, which does not cross-react in the cortisol assay.

Indications

To distinguish Cushing's disease from other causes of Cushing's syndrome.

Contraindications

As for the low-dose dexamethasone suppression test but in addition care should be exercised in patients with psychiatric manifestations of Cushing's syndrome, which may significantly worsen following higher doses of dexamethasone.

Practical details

Before investigation

This test should only be undertaken in individuals in whom the diagnosis of Cushing's syndrome has been confirmed. Ideally it should be performed as an inpatient.

The investigation

1 **Day 0**. 9.00 am. Take blood for serum cortisol
2 After venesection, give dexamethasone 2.0 mg orally every 6 h (i.e. at 9.00 am, 3.00 pm, 9.00 pm and 3.00 am) for 48 h
3 **Day 2**. 9.00 am. Take blood for serum cortisol (i.e. 6 h after last dose).

Note that some centres also routinely check serum cortisol after 24 h.

After investigation

Interpretation

Serum cortisol at completion of the test suppresses to ≤50% of the basal value in the majority of cases of Cushing's disease but not with other causes of Cushing's syndrome.

Complications

As with the low-dose test, complications are mainly restricted to the interpretation of results. Just as no single test can reliably confirm or refute the diagnosis of Cushing's syndrome, determination of the aetiology should not be based simply upon the result of one investigation. This is important with the high-dose dexamethasone suppression test, since approximately 10% of pituitary adenomas fail to suppress, whilst a smaller number of ectopic ACTH-secreting tumours do so.

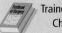
Trainer PJ, Besser M. *The Bart's Endocrine Protocols*, 1st edn. Churchill Livingstone, 1995.

3.2.3 ORAL GLUCOSE TOLERANCE TEST IN ACROMEGALY

Principle

GH secretion is pulsatile. As the hormone is rapidly cleared from the circulation, basal GH concentrations are undetectable most of the time. For these reasons, a single random blood sample is not a reliable assessment of GH secretion and dynamic tests are preferred. Normally, glucose suppresses GH secretion. In acromegaly, however, GH levels are paradoxically increased or not suppressed by glucose.

Indications

Patients with suspected acromegaly.

Contraindications

None.

Practical details

Before the investigation

Fast from midnight.

The investigation

1 Site an intravenous cannula
2 Take a basal blood sample for measurement of glucose and GH
3 Give 75 g of oral glucose (equivalent to approximately 390 mL of Lucozade®)
4 Take further blood samples for glucose and GH at 30, 60, 90 and 120 min.

After the investigation

Interpretation

Suppression of GH to less than 1 mU/L excludes the diagnosis of acromegaly. The glucose results may also show impaired glucose tolerance or DM, which can complicate acromegaly. Other conditions may give rise to non-suppressibility of GH after an oral glucose, but these are essentially catabolic conditions associated with high GH and low IGF-I levels and are unlikely to cause confusion in the clinical context.

 Duncan E, Wass JAH. Investigation protocol: acromegaly and its investigation. *Clin Endocrinol* 1999; 50: 285–293.

3.3 Other investigations

3.3.1 THYROID FUNCTION TESTS

Principle

There are a number of ways with which to assess the hypothalamo–pituitary–thyroid axis biochemically. Most laboratories routinely measure TSH levels, with many only going on to perform further thyroid function tests (TFTs) if they are specifically requested or indicated on the basis of an abnormal TSH result. Determination of FT_4 and FT_3 levels avoids many of the problems that are associated with interpreting the results of total hormone measurements.

Indications

TFTs are frequently requested, as hyper- and hypothyroidism are common diseases that may be difficult to diagnose clinically and are relatively easy to treat successfully.

Complications

There are a number of common pitfalls in the interpretation of TFTs.

'Sick euthyroid syndrome'

In non-thyroidal illness, concentrations of FT_3, FT_4 and TSH can all 'sag' at various times during the clinical course. In particular, hospitalized patients tend to have lower T_3 and higher reverse T_3 (rT_3) levels than healthy volunteers, due to reduced activity of the enzyme responsible for peripheral conversion of T_4 to T_3 and rT_3 to T_2.

 It is best not to test the thyroid function of ill patients unless there is clinical evidence of thyroid disease or concern that hyper- or hypothyroidism may be contributing to the patient's problems.

During thyrotoxicosis treatment

 Focus on the FT_4 levels shortly after beginning treatment for thyrotoxicosis, as the TSH may remain suppressed for weeks or months.

Pituitary disease

In clinically hypothyroid patients with a low FT_4 whose TSH is not elevated, consider the possibility of pituitary disease causing secondary hypothyroidism. Check remaining anterior pituitary function (hypopituitarism, see Section 2.1.7, p. 57), and remember that if there is evidence of cortisol deficiency, this must be corrected before thyroid replacement is instituted.

 In hypopituitary patients on T_4 replacement, remember to titrate the dose of T_4 against the FT_4 concentration: in this context it is probably safest to ignore the TSH.

Early pregnancy

In the first trimester of pregnancy, hCG secretion results in elevated concentrations of FT_4 and FT_3, and suppression of TSH. This is more marked in patients with hyperemesis gravidarum.

Drugs

Various drugs can interfere with thyroid function through one or more mechanisms:

• high doses of salicylates, furosemide (frusemide) or phenytoin may compete with hormone binding to thyroxine-binding globulin, resulting in increased free (but not total) hormone levels

• amiodarone, high-dose propranolol and oral cholecystographic agents inhibit peripheral conversion of T_4 to T_3

• dopamine, L-dopa and glucocorticoids may inhibit TSH secretion

• heparin increases FT_4 levels due to an *in vitro* assay artefact.

Chopra IJ. Euthyroid sick syndrome: is it a misnomer? *J Clin Endocrinol Metab* 1997; 82: 329–334.
Klee GG, Hay ID. Biochemical testing of thyroid function. *Endocrinol Metab Clin North Am* 1997; 26: 763–775.
Rae P, Farrar J, Beckett G, Toft A. Assessment of thyroid status in elderly people. *BMJ* 1993; 307: 177–180.

3.3.2 WATER DEPRIVATION TEST

Principle

In the presence of DI, water deprivation leads to intravascular depletion with an increase in plasma osmolality; urine osmolality remains inappropriately low due to a continued diuresis. In cranial DI (i.e. deficiency of ADH), administration of synthetic ADH (desmopressin [DDAVP]) corrects the defect to allow concentration of urine; by contrast, the urine remains dilute in nephrogenic DI (i.e. resistance to the action of ADH).

Indications

Diagnosis of DI and distinction from primary polydipsia.

Contraindications

• Suspected or confirmed thyroid and/or adrenal insufficiency. Ensure adequate hormone replacement prior to test

• Hypovolaemia.

Practical details

Before the investigation

Although fluid restriction is not necessary prior to the test, ask the patient to avoid excessive intake. Allow a light breakfast but no tea or coffee. Continue normal steroid replacement if the patient is receiving this.

The investigation

1 At 8.00 am, weigh the patient (with an empty bladder) and calculate 97% of this basal level
2 Under direct supervision, deprive the patient of all fluid and food for 8 h. Do not allow him/her to smoke
3 Measure and record all urine volumes on an hourly basis
4 Measure plasma and urine osmolalities at 0, 2, 4, 6 and 8 h
5 Weigh the patient at 2, 4, 6, 7 and 8 h
6 At the conclusion of the test, give desmopressin 2 µg i.m. and continue collecting urine samples and measuring urine osmolalities for a further 4 h. Allow the patient to drink and eat freely during this period.

If at any point during the test there is a greater than 3% drop in weight compared to the basal level, check plasma osmolality urgently. If this has risen to >295 mosmol/kg, give desmopressin 2 µg i.m. and allow the patient to drink. Otherwise consider continuing the test under close supervision. Abandon if the patient loses ≥5% of body weight.

After the investigation

Interpretation

• In normal subjects, plasma osmolality increases but remains below 295 mosmol/kg; urine osmolality rises as urine volume falls

• With cranial DI, urine osmolality fails to rise and a relative diuresis continues despite the increasing plasma osmolality. Following desmopressin, the urine concentrates normally

• Nephrogenic DI is similar to cranial DI, except that there is a failure of urine concentration in response to desmopressin

• With primary polydipsia, excessive fluid intake prior to the test may result in an apparent continued diuresis despite fluid restriction. Plasma osmolality remains below 295 mosmol/kg.

Trainer PJ, Besser M. *The Bart's Endocrine Protocols*, 1st edn. Churchill Livingstone, 1995.

4 Self-assessment

Answers on pp. 135–141.

Question 1

In the investigation and management of hyponatraemia (T/F):

A Venlafaxine is a recognized cause of the syndrome of inappropriate ADH secretion (SIADH)

B Hypertonic saline should be given if the sodium is less than 120 mmol/L

C The cause can be readily identified on the basis of simple biochemical tests

D Measurement of ADH levels is helpful

E Lithium may be used to treat SIADH.

Question 2

Primary hyperparathyroidism (T/F):

A Is a recognized cause of osteoporosis

B Leads to enhanced intestinal calcium absorption

C Complicates chronic renal failure

D Is excluded if the PTH level is not elevated

E Is associated with hypertension.

Question 3

Topic: salt and water balance

A Cranial diabetes insipidus

B Primary hyperaldosteronism

C Syndrome of inappropriate ADH secretion (SIADH)

D Nephrogenic diabetes insipidus

E Psychogenic polydipsia

F Hyporeninaemic hypoaldosteronism.

Select the disorder of salt and water balance which is most commonly associated with each of the following conditions.

1 Recurrent pyelonephritis
2 Bronchogenic carcinoma
3 Hypercalcaemia
4 Adrenal adenoma
5 Histiocytosis X.

Question 4

Which of the following statements are true?

A The multiple endocrine neoplasia (MEN) type 1 syndrome is characterized by parathyroid hyperplasia, pancreatic tumours and phaeochromocytoma

B An elevated proinsulin : insulin ratio is found in patients with insulinoma

C ACE inhibitors are a recognized cause of hypoglycaemia

D Ectopic insulin secretion by retroperitoneal sarcomas commonly leads to fasting hypoglycaemia

E Selective intra-arterial injection of calcium may aid angiographic localization of an insulinoma.

Question 5

Genetic haemochromatosis (T/F):

A Is inherited in an autosomal dominant manner with incomplete penetrance

B Always arises as a consequence of mutations in the HFE gene

C May present with intractable heart failure

D Does not present before the age of 30 years

E Only requires treatment by venesection once symptoms develop.

Question 6

Which of the following statements are true regarding the investigation of acromegaly?

A MRI commonly reveals evidence of a pituitary macroadenoma

B Suppression of growth hormone (GH) levels following an oral glucose tolerance test confirms the diagnosis

C GH levels are elevated whilst insulin-like growth factor-1 (IGF-1) levels are suppressed

D Hypergonadotrophic hypogonadism is a common finding

E A low random GH level excludes the diagnosis of acromegaly.

Question 7

Topic: investigation of Cushing's syndrome

A Low-dose dexamethasone suppression test

B Inferior petrosal sinus sampling following corticotrophin releasing hormone (CRH) stimulation

C Insulin tolerance test

D CT of thorax

E 24-h urinary free cortisol (UFC) estimation

F CT of adrenal glands.

For each clinical scenario shown, select the next investigation of choice from those listed above:

1 Distinction between true Cushing's and pseudo-Cushing's syndrome

2 Suspected Cushing's disease in an individual with abnormal low-dose dexamethasone suppression and loss of diurnal cortisol secretion

3 Confirmed Cushing's syndrome with suppressed plasma ACTH levels

4 Failure of suppression of serum cortisol following high-dose dexamethasone with no central to peripheral ACTH gradient on inferior petrosal sinus sampling.

Question 8

In the United Kingdom, osteomalacia (T/F):
A Is rarely seen outside the Asian community
B May present with pathological hip fracture
C Due to malabsorption requires parenteral vitamin D
D Due to X-linked hypophosphataemia requires no follow up
E May complicate the management of tuberculosis.

Question 9

Regarding the metabolic syndrome (T/F):
A Impaired glucose tolerance is of no consequence
B Low birth weight is a recognized association
C Fibrinogen levels are typically elevated
D Levels of small, dense low density lipoproteins (LDL) are reduced
E An increased prevalence amongst South Asians in the UK is recognized.

Question 10

A previously fit 40-year-old man is referred for further investigation of his hypertension, which has been refractory to treatment with bendrofluazide. Twenty-four-hour ambulatory blood pressure monitoring has confirmed a mean value of 180/100. The lower pole of the right kidney is palpable on abdominal examination, and there is evidence of Grade II hypertensive retinopathy on fundoscopy. A number of screening tests have been performed by his GP:
• Urea and electrolytes: Na^+ 129 mmol/L, K^+ 2.8 mmol/L, urea 6.0 mmol/L, creatinine 104 μmol/L
• Corrected calcium: 2.40 mmol/L
• TSH: 1.5 mU/L
• Urinalysis: negative
• UFC: 120 nmol/24 h
• ECG and CXR: within normal limits.
Which of the following statements are true?
A Hyponatraemia makes the diagnosis of primary hyper-aldosteronism unlikely
B The addition of an ACE inhibitor should be recommended
C Cushing's syndrome has been reliably excluded
D Polycystic kidney disease is likely given the clinical findings
E Hyponatraemia should be corrected with fludrocortisone.

Question 11

From the following list, select the most likely diagnosis in a 55-year-old male given the MRI appearances shown in Fig. 62.
A Cushing's disease
B Lymphocytic hypophysitis
C Histiocytosis X

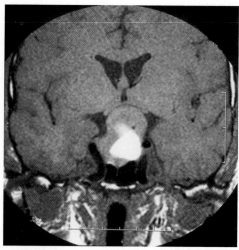

Fig. 62 Question 11.

D Non-functioning pituitary adenoma
E Sheehan's syndrome.

Question 12

Which of the following features favour a diagnosis of type 2 rather than type 1 diabetes mellitus?
A Presence of antibodies to islet cells
B Association with other autoimmune diseases
C Onset later in life
D Proneness to ketosis
E Increased body mass index.

Question 13

A 35-year-old type 1 diabetic is found to have micro-albuminuria. Which of the following statements are true?
A He is at higher risk of developing diabetic retinopathy
B Measurement of urea and electrolytes is likely to reveal evidence of renal impairment, and the glomerular filtration rate will be reduced
C ACE inhibitors are useful even in the absence of hypertension
D The risk of macrovascular complications remains unchanged
E Good diabetic control does not influence the renal outcome once microalbuminuria is present.

Question 14

Which of the following are associated with hypogonado-trophic hypogonadism?
A Colour blindness
B Premature ovarian failure
C XXY karyotype
D Large testes
E Cryptorchidism.

Question 15

Which set of thyroid function tests in Table 62 are most likely to correlate with the clinical scenarios outlined below?

Table 62 Question 15.

	TSH (mU/L)	FT4 (pmol/L)
Normal ranges	0.5–5	10–25
A	<0.5	20
B	20	
C	1	7
D	2	20
E	<0.5	40
F	12	15

1 A patient presenting with unintentional weight loss and palpitations

2 A patient treated with radioiodine for thyrotoxicosis 6 months ago, who has gained 5 kg in weight

3 A patient who was found to have primary hypothyroidism 4 weeks ago, and was started on thyroxine 100 µg once daily immediately

4 A patient who had radiotherapy to the pituitary fossa 5 years ago, and has recently developed tiredness and lethargy

5 A patient who was started on treatment with carbimazole for thyrotoxicosis 4 weeks ago, and is now clinically euthyroid.

Question 16

Regarding Turner's syndrome (T/F):

A The diagnosis is unlikely in girls who do not exhibit the classical features

B You should take care to explain to patients that they are only half female

C Spontaneous puberty may occur

D Short stature is the result of growth hormone deficiency

E Affected women usually have a normal IQ.

Question 17

Topic: treatment of endocrine conditions

A Bromocriptine

B Hydrocortisone

C Carbamazepine

D Testosterone

E Desmopressin (DDAVP)

F Oestrogen with progestogen hormone replacement therapy

G Carbimazole

H Fludrocortisone

I Sildenafil ('Viagra').

Select the most appropriate drug treatment (A–I) for each of the following:

1 A patient presenting with Graves' disease

2 A patient presenting with an Addisonian crisis

3 A 40-year-old patient with diabetes and erectile dysfunction

4 A patient with infertility caused by a microprolactinoma

5 A patient with central diabetes insipidus

6 A 40-year-old patient with Kallmann's syndrome and erectile dysfunction.

Question 18

Regarding gynaecomastia (T/F):

A Hyperthyroidism is a recognized cause

B It is a recognized finding in body builders

C It frequently complicates treatment with amiodarone

D In pubertal boys, it suggests an underlying testicular or adrenal tumour

E It is associated with chronic obstructive pulmonary disease.

Question 19

Possible causes of hyperprolactinaemia include:

A Treatment with dopamine agonists

B A non-functioning pituitary adenoma

C Hyperthyroidism

D Foreplay

E Venepuncture.

Question 20

Regarding the polycystic ovarian syndrome (PCOS) (T/F):

A Oligomenorrhoea is associated with a risk of osteoporosis

B A pelvic ultrasound scan demonstrating polycystic ovaries is highly suggestive of the condition

C Insulin resistance is a recognized association

D Hormonal treatment of hirsutism should not be attempted whilst the patient is trying to conceive

E Mechanical hair removal increases re-growth.

Question 21

Topic: endocrine investigations

A Serum prolactin concentration

B CT head scan

C Growth hormone levels during an insulin tolerance test

D Short synacthen test

E 24-h urine collection for 5-hydroxyindoleacetic acid (5HIAA)

F CT scan of the abdomen

G Pregnancy test

H MRI scan of the pituitary fossa

I Growth hormone levels during an oral glucose tolerance test

J 24-h urine collection for catecholamines.

Select the most appropriate initial investigation for each of the following patients:

1 A 60-year-old woman presenting with persistent facial flushing and diarrhoea

2 A 20-year-old woman presenting with a 3-month history of amenorrhoea

3 A 50-year-old man with type 2 diabetes, hypertension and osteoarthritis, referred by his GP for sleep studies and a second carpal tunnel release

4 A 40-year-old man with erectile dysfunction, found by his GP to have normal renal function, liver function and thyroid function, but a prolactin concentration elevated at 1300 mU/L and 1500 mU/L on two separate occasions (normal range <200 mU/L)

5 A 30-year-old woman appropriately treated with hydrocortisone, thyroxine and sex hormone replacement therapy following pituitary radiotherapy in childhood, presenting with a chronic lack of energy, poor exercise tolerance and low mood.

Question 22

Regarding the carcinoid syndrome (T/F):

A Complete resection of a primary gastrointestinal carcinoid tumour may be curative in a patient with carcinoid syndrome

B A 24-h urine collection for 5-hydroxytryptophan (5-HT) is a useful diagnostic test

C Tumours may express somatostatin receptors

D Octreotide therapy is associated with an increased tendency to renal stone formation

E Patients do not usually live for more than a few months once liver metastases are present.

Question 23

In Addison's disease (T/F):

A Associated vitiligo leads to skin pigmentation

B Patients should be advised to take their evening dose of hydrocortisone last thing at night with a snack

C An autoimmune basis is not excluded by the failure to detect adrenal autoantibodies

D The diagnosis should always be confirmed with a Synacthen test prior to instituting treatment

E Patients should be advised to alter their steroid dose if they are ill without first seeking medical advice.

Question 24

Topic: endocrine drug side effects

A Glibenclamide

B Amiodarone

C Desmopressin (DDAVP)

D Bromocriptine

E Metoclopramide

F Carbimazole

G Alfacalcidol.

Match the drugs (A–G) to the potential side effects:

1 Nausea, vomiting and dizziness

2 Neutropaenia

3 Hypoglycaemia

4 Galactorrhoea

5 Thyroid dysfunction

6 Hyponatraemia.

Question 25

Topic: erectile dysfunction (T/F):

A Is uncommon in men who do not have diabetes

B Is unlikely to be due to underlying organic pathology if the patient still experiences early-morning erections

C Is unlikely to respond to sildenafil ('Viagra') if a spontaneous erection does not occur within 60 min of taking the maximum 100 mg dose

D Is commonly improved by testosterone therapy

E May arise as a consequence of hyperprolactinaemia.

Question 26

Regarding pituitary hormone replacement therapy (T/F):

A Hypopituitary patients treated with testosterone must be warned that this is likely to restore their fertility

B Patients treated for diabetes insipidus with desmopressin should increase their dose to cover intercurrent illnesses

C Hydrocortisone treatment should be started before concurrent hypothyroidism is treated

D Men who are not sexually active do not require testosterone replacement if they do not want it

E The combined oral contraceptive pill is the best way to provide oestrogen replacement therapy for hypopituitary women who have not had a hysterectomy.

Question 27

A 22-year-old woman with headaches and galactorrhoea is noted to have a mildly elevated prolactin level at 950 mU/L (normal up to 400 mU/L). An MRI scan of her pituitary fossa is shown in Fig. 63. The appearances are those of:

A A normal pituitary gland

B A microprolactinoma

C A macroprolactinoma

D A non-functioning adenoma compressing the pituitary stalk

E Pituitary apoplexy.

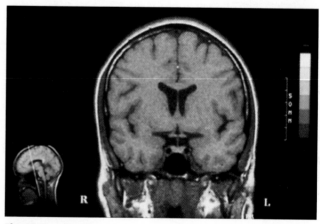

Fig. 63 Question 27.

Question 28

Regarding constitutional delay of puberty (T/F):

A In general, it is not necessary to investigate or treat suspected cases before 16 years of age

B Treatment with sex steroids will inhibit the natural onset of puberty

C The growth spurt typically happens before the child enters puberty

D There may be a family history

E Affected children will usually achieve their predicted adult height.

Question 29

A 52-year-old male has been attending the diabetes clinic for 3 years and is currently on gliclazide 80 mg b.d. At annual review he is noted to have background retinopathy, dipstick positive microalbuminuria and 2-finger-breadth hepatomegaly. The results of subsequent investigations are as follows:

- HbA_{1c} 7.9%
- Urea   4.5 mmol/L
- Creatinine   110 μmol/L
- ALT   320 IU/L (normal <50 IU/L)
- Alkaline phosphatase 150 IU/L (normal <120 IU/L)
- Albumin   42 g/L
- INR   1.2
- Hepatitis A, B, C serology negative

Which condition should be excluded?

Which non-invasive investigation would help to confirm your diagnosis?

What treatment should be recommended?

Question 30

A 65-year-old obese type 2 diabetic, who has failed to attend for follow up during the last 5 years, is referred by his GP for review of his diabetes and for consideration for treatment with sildenafil ('Viagra'). On examination, he is noted to be hypertensive (150/90 mmHg), with absent peripheral pulses. Fundoscopy reveals the appearances shown in Fig. 64. Which of the following statements are true?

A Urgent referral to an ophthalmologist is indicated

B The retinal appearances are suggestive of advanced hypertensive retinopathy

C Insulin treatment should be recommended to aid weight loss

D Treatment with a β-blocker should be avoided

E Sildenafil can be safely prescribed provided the patient is not currently receiving treatment with a nitrate.

Question 31

Which of the following statements are true regarding hypothyroidism in pregnancy?

A Thyroid hormone requirements typically decrease in the third trimester

B There is a higher risk of congenital malformations, miscarriages and stillbirths in untreated mothers

C Maternal TSH levels should be suppressed to prevent the development of thyrotoxicosis in the fetus

D T_3 (triiodothyronine) is the preferred form of thyroid hormone replacement

E Subacute thyroiditis is the commonest underlying cause.

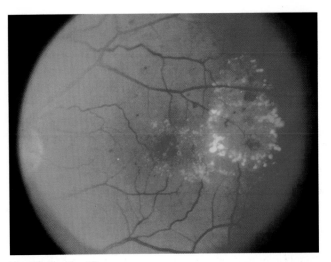

Fig. 64 Question 30.

Question 32

A 44-year-old man presents with a 3-month history of headaches, fatigue and generalized weakness. He has recently been found to be hypothyroid by his GP and started on thyroxine 100 μg/day, but with little change in his symptoms. The following investigations were undertaken following his referral to hospital:

- Free T_4 22.5 pmol/L (normal 9–20 pmol/L)
- TSH   0.10 mU/L (normal 0.4–4 mU/L)

Short synacthen test:
- 0′ cortisol   135 nmol/L
- 30′ cortisol   275 nmol/L

Oral glucose tolerance test (OGTT) (Table 63)

A In addition to hypothyroidism, list three other diagnoses suggested by these results.

B What other abnormalities of pituitary function might you expect to find?

Table 63 Question 32.

Time (min)	Glucose (mmol/L)	Growth hormone (mU/L)
0	7.8	22.5
30	–	24.5
60	–	22.0
90	–	20.2
120	12.8	18.6

Question 33

Which of the following investigations are often useful in discriminating the ectopic ACTH syndrome from pituitary dependent Cushing's disease?

A Insulin tolerance test (ITT)

B Corticotrophin releasing hormone (CRH) test

C Selective venous sampling for ACTH

D Low-dose dexamethasone suppression test

E Urea and electrolytes

Question 34

A 70-year-old woman presents to her GP with palpitations and shortness of breath. On examination she is noted to be in atrial fibrillation with warm peripheries and a fine resting tremor. Her GP is somewhat surprised to find the following thyroid function tests:

- Free T_4 18 pmol/L (normal 9–20 pmol/L)
- TSH   <0.03 mU/L (normal 0.4–4 mU/L)

A What further test would you request?
B What is the most likely diagnosis?
C How would you confirm the diagnosis?
D What treatment would you recommend?

Question 35

Amenorrhoea is often found in the setting of (T/F):

A Klinefelter's syndrome
B Turner's syndrome
C Hyperprolactinaemia
D Hypothyroidism
E Anorexia nervosa.

Question 36

A 29-year-old woman complains of excessive weight gain since the birth of her second child 2 years ago, despite repeated attempts to diet. Her only regular medication is the oral contraceptive pill. Her body mass index is calculated to be 35 kg/m². The remainder of the physical examination is unremarkable. The results of initial investigations are as follows:

- Free T_4 15 pmol/L (normal 9–20 pmol/L)
- TSH   1.2 mU/L (normal 0.4–4 mU/L)
- Urea and   Within normal limits
  electrolytes
- Fasting glucose   4.6 mmol/l
  Overnight dexamethasone suppression test:
- 09.00 am cortisol   <50 nmol/L

What is the most likely cause for this woman's weight gain? What treatment would you recommend?

Question 37

A 42-year-old woman with a 6-month history of tiredness and lethargy is admitted as an emergency complaining of a severe retro-orbital headache and visual disturbance (Fig. 65). The results of an urgent MRI scan are shown in Fig. 66. The appearances are most in keeping with:

A Pituitary apoplexy complicated by a sixth nerve palsy
B Craniopharyngioma and an associated pupillary sparing 3rd nerve palsy
C Lymphocytic hypophysitis with suprasellar extension
D Acromegaly with lateral extension into the left cavernous sinus
E Subarachnoid haemorrhage due to a posterior communicating artery aneurysm
F Pituitary apoplexy complicated by a complete 3rd nerve palsy.

Question 38

An obese 46-year-old man with hypertension is noted to

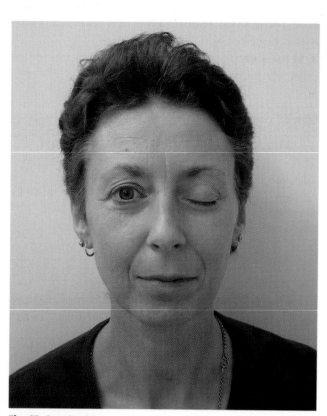

Fig. 65 Question 37.

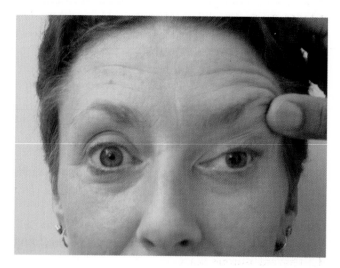

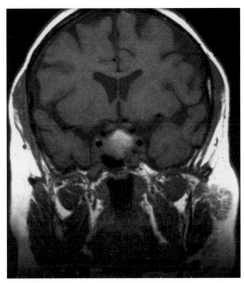

Fig. 66 Question 37.

have glycosuria during a routine check up. His GP has organized an oral glucose tolerance test (OGTT) (Table 64).

The patient should be advised that (T/F):

A The OGTT shows evidence of impaired glucose tolerance

B He has unfortunately developed type 2 diabetes

C He requires treatment with metformin

D The results of the OGTT are normal

E Weight loss is necessary.

Table 64 Question 38.

Time (min)	Plasma glucose (mmol/L)
0	5.6
60	9.9
120	6.6

Question 39

Regarding thyrotoxicosis (T/F):

A The finding of lid lag and lid retraction is suggestive of Graves' disease

B Long-term treatment with carbimazole is the preferred option in the case of a solitary toxic adenoma

C Thyroid isotope scans are useful in differentiating thyroiditis from Graves' disease

D Radioiodine therapy should not be offered to patients less than 50 years of age

E Treatment with amiodarone is a recognized cause.

Question 40

A 60-year-old man presents with confusion and a preceding history of polyuria and polydipsia. Initial investigations show normal renal function, but the serum calcium is elevated at 3.6 mmol/L with a serum phosphate of 1.6 mmol/L and a markedly raised erythrocyte sedimentation rate (90 mm/h).

A What is the most likely cause of the hypercalcaemia?

B What further tests should be performed, and why?

C What treatment should be initiated?

Question 41

Topic: osteoporosis (T/F):

A Rarely affects men

B May complicate long-standing hyperthyroidism

C May cause pain in the absence of fractures

D Should only be treated once fracture has occurred

E Should always be treated with calcium supplements.

Question 42

Topic: hyperlipidaemia

A Lipoprotein lipase deficiency

B Nephrotic syndrome

C Homozygous familial hypercholesterolaemia

D Familial combined hyperlipidaemia

E Alcoholic cirrhosis

F Type III hyperlipoproteinaemia

G Primary biliary cirrhosis.

For each clinical scenario outlined below, select the most likely diagnosis from those listed above.

1 Tendon xanthomata in a 15 year old

2 Jaundice and xanthelasmata in a 60-year-old woman

3 Marked mixed hyperlipidaemia in a patient whose parents are known to have normal lipid profiles

4 Hyperlipidaemia resistant to all drug treatment in a patient with peripheral oedema.

Question 43

A Bendrofluazide

B Atenolol

C Methyldopa

D Erythromycin

E Rifampicin

F Penicillin

G Aspirin

H Paracetamol

I Diclofenac sodium

J Pethidine

K Metformin

L Sulphonylureas.

For each of the following situations, select from the drugs listed above those that may safely be given to a patient with acute intermittent porphyria. Note: there may be more than one agent that is safe, in which case all possible options should be listed.

1 Hypertension

2 Infection

3 Analgesia

4 Diabetes mellitus.

Question 44

A 12-year-old girl presents with polyuria, weight loss and recurrent skin infections.

A What is the most likely diagnosis, and how would you confirm it?

B What is known of the aetiology of this condition?

C How should she be treated?

Question 45

Topic: management of diabetes mellitus

A A low-carbohydrate, low-fat diet

B Gliclazide

C Metformin

D Insulin

E Lisinopril

F Atenolol

G Pravastatin.

For each of the situations described below, select the most appropriate treatment from those listed above.

1 A newly diagnosed type 2 diabetic

2 An obese type 2 diabetic with an HbA_{1C} >8% despite dietary modification

3 A diabetic with persistent microalbuminuria

4 A diabetic with a blood pressure of 150/95 mmHg and a history of erectile dysfunction.

Answers to Self-assessment

Answers to Question 1

T, F, F, F, T

A Tricyclic antidepressants are a well recognized cause of SIADH, but it is now clear that the newer selective serotonin reuptake inhibitors (SSRIs), such as venlafaxine, may also cause SIADH.

B Hypertonic saline is a potentially dangerous treatment and should only be given where there is evidence of encephalopathy; the sodium concentration is irrelevant.

C The cause of hyponatraemia, and particularly the diagnosis of SIADH, cannot be established through biochemical tests alone.

D Isolated measurement of ADH levels is not helpful, as ADH is influenced by many factors in addition to plasma osmolality.

E Lithium, like demeclocycline, induces nephrogenic diabetes insipidus and can be used to treat SIADH when other measures fail; its use is limited by unwanted side effects.

Answers to Question 2

T, T, F, F, T

A Primary hyperparathyroidism causes osteoclast activation and may therefore lead to secondary osteoporosis.

B PTH stimulates 1α hydroxylation of $25(OH)D_3$ and the resulting $1,25(OH)_2D_3$ stimulates intestinal calcium absorption.

C Primary hyperparathyroidism is associated with both urolithiasis and nephrocalcinosis, which may result in renal failure; secondary hyperparathyroidism is an appropriate response to the hypocalcaemia of renal failure; tertiary hyperparathyroidism denotes the development of autonomous parathyroid function.

D Serum PTH should be suppressed in hypercalcaemia; absence of suppression is the hallmark of hyperparathyroidism, and the level may lie within the normal range.

E Hypertension is a recognized feature of isolated primary hyperparathyroidism. In addition, it may reflect a coexistent phaeochromocytoma in the setting of the multiple endocrine neoplasia type 2 syndromes.

Answers to Question 3

1D 2C 3D 4B 5A

1 Recurrent pyelonephritis may lead to damage to the renal medulla with consequent loss of formation of a concentration gradient, such that urine passing through the collecting ducts cannot be concentrated.

2 Bronchogenic carcinoma is a recognized cause of ectopic ADH secretion.

3 Hypercalcaemia and hypokalaemia both reduce urinary concentrating capacity.

4 Benign adrenal adenomas account for approximately 75% of cases of primary hyperaldosteronism (Conn's syndrome).

5 Cranial diabetes insipidus and anterior pituitary insufficiency may be the presenting features of Histiocytosis X.

Hyporeninaemic hypoaldosteronism typically occurs in elderly patients with diabetes and mild renal insufficiency. It is usually discovered incidentally on routine screening, manifesting as hyperkalaemia and acidosis. Following exclusion of other causes of hyperkalaemia, it may be treated with fludrocortisone (0.05 mg/day).

Answers to Question 4

F, T, T, F, T

A Parathyroid, Pituitary and Pancreatic—the '3 Ps' of MEN type 1 (Section 2.7, p. 115).

B In normal subjects, proinsulin contributes <20% of the total measured insulin immunoreactivity. This ratio is usually significantly increased in patients with insulinoma.

C ACE inhibitors (ACE-I) increase sensitivity to insulin and can theoretically potentiate the risk of hypoglycaemia in insulin or sulphonylurea-treated diabetics. However, this is rarely a problem in clinical practice, and should not preclude their use, given the number of potential benefits which they confer in this high-risk population.

D A number of non-pancreatic tumours may be associated with fasting hypoglycaemia (e.g. retroperitoneal sarcoma, hepatoma). Several mechanisms are likely to contribute to this, including release of peptides with insulin-like action. True ectopic insulin secretion appears to be very rare.

E Unlike normal islet cells, insulinomas release insulin in response to calcium stimulation. Simultaneous venous sampling following selective intra-arterial calcium injection has been reported to help localize small tumours not easily seen using other techniques.

Answers to Question 5

F, F, T, F, F

A Genetic haemochromatosis is recessively inherited. Some older textbooks state that it is inherited dominantly with incomplete penetrance; this confusion arose from the high gene frequency (~5%) which allows a reasonably high probability of heterozygote–homozygote pairings with all offspring affected (an apparent dominant pattern).

B Neonatal and juvenile genetic haemochromatosis are not due to mutations in the HFE gene, and even 10% of adult haemochromatosis patients do not have the common HFE mutation.

C Haemochromatosis can give rise to a dilated cardiomyopathy; it is important to recognize this condition since it may respond to reduction of iron overload through venesection.

D Although haemochromatosis does not usually present until after 40 years of age, more rapidly progressive forms even of adult genetic haemochromatosis are recognized.

E Venesection should be started once iron overload has been diagnosed, to help prevent the development of complications.

Answers to Question 6

T, F, F, F, F

A Approximately 75% of cases of acromegaly are due to a pituitary macroadenoma (>1 cm in diameter).

B Failure of GH levels to suppress during an oral glucose tolerance test (OGTT—Section 3.2.3, p. 122) is the characteristic biochemical hallmark of acromegaly.

C Elevated GH levels stimulate IGF-1 release, which is responsible for the typical soft tissue changes and organomegaly.

D Hypogonadotrophic hypogonadism reflects suppression of gonadotroph activity by tumour expansion and hyperprolactinaemia.

E A single low GH level does not rule out acromegaly since GH secretion is pulsatile. Although repeatedly low levels argue against the diagnosis, formal exclusion requires the demonstration of normal GH suppression during an OGTT. IGF-1 levels may be helpful in monitoring response to therapy.

Answers to Question 7

1C 2B 3F 4D

1 The cortisol response to insulin-induced hypoglycaemia is preserved in pseudo-Cushing's syndrome, contrasting with the subnormal response typically seen in true Cushing's syndrome.

2 The sensitivity of inferior petrosal sampling is improved following CRH stimulation. In a patient with Cushing's syndrome, an ACTH ratio of ≥2 between inferior petrosal and peripheral samples is strongly suggestive of a pituitary source of ACTH.

3 In the absence of exogenous corticosteroid use, adrenal causes of ACTH independent Cushing's syndrome must be distinguished.

4 Failure of suppression of serum cortisol following high-dose dexamethasone, with no detectable ACTH gradient on inferior petrosal sinus sampling is strongly suggestive of ectopic ACTH secretion. Small cell carcinoma of the lung and bronchial carcinoids account for >50% of cases.

Answers to Question 8

F, T, F, F, T

A Whilst osteomalacia is more frequent among Asian immigrants to the UK, it is still common among the elderly indigenous population where reduced exposure to sunlight and dietary vitamin D deficiency often coincide.

B Although the pathognomonic radiological feature of osteomalacia is the pseudofracture, osteomalacic bone is weak and prone to true fracture as well.

C Parenteral vitamin D may be used in malabsorption, but usually there is sufficient absorption of the vitamin D metabolite alfacalcidol to avoid the need for intramuscular injections.

D X-linked hypophosphataemia requires monitoring, both of the phosphate supplements required in this condition (and other hypophosphataemic causes of osteomalacia) and for the complication of spinal stenosis due to new bone formation.

E Tuberculosis does not cause osteomalacia directly (although it is more common in some groups who are prone to vitamin D deficiency), but it is treated with prolonged courses of the enzyme-inducing antibiotic rifampicin, which increases vitamin D clearance and may thereby cause vitamin D deficient osteomalacia.

Answers to Question 9

F, T, T, F, T

A Impaired glucose tolerance, whether as part of the metabolic syndrome or not, carries an increased risk of macrovascular disease.

B The reported association of the features of the metabolic syndrome with low birth weight are thought to reflect poor maternal nutrition during pregnancy (the Barker hypothesis).

C, D High levels of fibrinogen and of the particularly atherogenic small, dense LDL particles are both features of the metabolic syndrome, although often not routinely measured in clinical practice.

E The metabolic syndrome is particularly common in South Asians in the UK and is thought to explain at least some of the increased risk of ischaemic heart disease in this community.

Answers to Question 10

F, F, F, F, F

A, B The existence of hypertension in a relatively young male should prompt consideration of secondary causes (see Case history 1.18). Hyponatraemia may reflect treatment with bendrofluazide and therefore does not exclude primary hyperaldosteronism. Ideally measurement of serum electrolytes and assessment of the renin–angiotensin–aldosterone system should be performed off all treatment, or if necessary whilst on agents which do not interfere directly with this axis, e.g. α-blockers.

C A single normal 24-h UFC collection does not reliably exclude Cushing's syndrome.

D The lower pole of the right kidney may be palpable in normal individuals.

E Hyponatraemia is likely to correct with cessation of the diuretic. There is little to suggest mineralocorticoid deficiency, which is usually associated with hypotension. Fludrocortisone is likely to severely exacerbate the pre-existing hypertension.

Answers to Question 11

D

The appearances are those of a pituitary macroadenoma with suprasellar extension. The high signal seen within the tumour represents an area of haemorrhage. Cushing's disease is most commonly due to a corticotroph micro-adenoma. Although lymphocytic hypophysitis may be indistinguishable from a pituitary macroadenoma, it is most commonly seen in pregnancy or the late postpartum period with only a small number of cases described in males. Histiocytosis X is a rare disorder characterized by histiocytic infiltration of multiple organs including, in some cases, both the anterior and posterior pituitary gland. Hypotension complicating postpartum haemorrhage may lead to hypopituitarism as a consequence of pituitary infarction, so-called Sheehan's syndrome.

Answers to Question 12

F, F, T, F, T

Type 2 diabetes (previously known as maturity-onset diabetes or non-insulin dependent diabetes) is strongly familial and usually affects relatively older individuals, although no age is exempt. It has a strong association with obesity: a BMI of >35 kg/m^2 increases the risk by 40-fold as compared with a BMI of <23 kg/m^2.

Type 1 diabetes (previously known as juvenile-onset or insulin-dependent diabetes) typically presents at a younger age. Genetic susceptibility interacts with environmental factors to predispose to autoimmune mediated destruction of pancreatic β cells. It is associated with other organ-specific autoimmune disorders including autoimmune thyroid disease, Addison's disease and pernicious anaemia. Type 1 diabetics are truly insulin dependent and prone to ketosis.

Answers to Question 13

T, F, T, F, F

A, D The presence of microalbuminuria is associated with both micro- and macrovascular complications in type 1 diabetes. Retinopathy is a microvascular complication and the presence of microalbuminuria denotes a higher risk for its development and/or progression.

B Renal function is usually preserved in the microalbuminuric and early stages (intermittent and early persistent proteinuria) of diabetic nephropathy.

C ACE inhibitors are useful in halting or slowing down the progression of microalbuminuria to overt nephropathy, even in the absence of hypertension, and should be prescribed provided there are no contraindications to their use.

E Good diabetic and blood pressure control are essential to halt or slow the progression of renal damage once micro-albuminuria is present.

Answers to Question 14

T, F, F, F, T

A, E Hypogonadotrophic hypogonadism denotes hypogonadism secondary to a hypothalamic or pituitary disorder. Kallmann's syndrome is characterized by hyposmia/anosmia, colour blindness, small soft testes and cryptorchidism, together with other features of hypogonadism.

B, C Premature ovarian failure and Klinefelter's syndrome (XXY) are associated with hypergonadotrophic hypogonadism (primary hypogonadism).

D Large testes are a feature of the Fragile X syndrome, which is associated with mental retardation.

Answers to Question 15

1E 2B 3F 4C 5A

1 Weight loss and palpitations are common manifestations of hyperthyroidism, which is associated with elevated free thyroid hormone levels in the presence of a suppressed TSH.

2 Radioiodine therapy predisposes to primary hypothyroidism with consequent increased pituitary TSH secretion.

3 Remember that following treatment for hypothyroidism, there is typically a lag phase before the TSH falls back into the normal range. Accordingly, the dose of thyroxine should be titrated against the free thyroid hormone concentration.

4 Although the FT$_4$ is low, the TSH is not elevated: together with the history, this suggests secondary hypothyroidism (in future, the TSH concentration should be ignored).

5 TSH usually remains suppressed for some time after commencing therapy for hyperthyroidism; therefore again, aim to titrate treatment to the free thyroid hormone concentration.

Answers to Question 16

F, F, T, F, T

A The karyotype of all girls with short stature and delayed puberty should be determined as the classical stigmata of Turner's syndrome may not be present.

B Quite the opposite! Patients should be reassured about their gender identification.

C True, but rare.

D This is not a growth hormone deficient condition, although growth hormone therapy may be used to try to maximize the final adult height.

E An important point, which is often not appreciated.

Answers to Question 17

1G 2B 3I 4A 5E 6D

1 Carbimazole and propylthiouracil are both suitable for the treatment of Graves' disease.

2 Intravenous hydrocortisone (100 mg stat) must be given without delay.

3 Sildenafil may improve sexual function in males with erectile dysfunction due to long-standing diabetes.

4 Suppression of the serum prolactin level back into the normal range may restore fertility.

5 Desmopressin is an effective treatment for cranial diabetes insipidus.

6 Kallmann's syndrome is characterized by hypogonadotrophic hypogonadism.

Answers to Question 18
T, T, F, F, F

B It can be associated with the abuse of anabolic steroids.

C It is a recognized side effect of many drugs, including digoxin and spironolactone, but not amiodarone (liver failure secondary to amiodarone, with subsequent gynaecomastia is likely to be very rare!).

D Gynaecomastia is frequently physiological/idiopathic in this age group.

E Both chronic liver disease and chronic renal failure are associated with gynaecomastia, but it is not a feature of chronic obstructive pulmonary disease *per se*.

Answers to Question 19
F, T, F, T, T

A, B Prolactin release is under tonic inhibitory control by dopamine. Pressure on the pituitary stalk may interrupt this regulatory pathway, thereby leading to hyperprolactinaemia, so-called stalk disconnection syndrome. Accordingly, dopamine agonists are used as medical therapy for hyperprolactinaemia.

C Hypothyroidism can lead to hyperprolactinaemia as a consequence of the trophic effects of hypothalamic TRH on prolactin release.

D, E Nipple stimulation may cause galactorrhoea long after breast-feeding has been discontinued. Stress (e.g. needle phobia) may lead to mild hyperprolactinaemia.

Answers to Question 20
F, F, T, T, F

A PCOS is not an oestrogen-deficient state.

B Many women who do not have PCOS have polycystic ovaries on ultrasound scanning.

C The 'metabolic form' of PCOS is associated with insulin resistance.

D Hormonal treatment involves either the combined oral contraceptive pill or the antiandrogen cyproterone acetate which is teratogenic.

E This is a myth.

Answers to Question 21
1E 2G 3I 4H 5C

1 Flushing and diarrhoea should prompt consideration of the carcinoid syndrome.

2 Do not get caught out!

3 The patient may have acromegaly—the biochemical diagnosis should precede radiological imaging; an insulin-like growth factor-1 concentration should also be checked.

4 A non-functioning pituitary tumour must be excluded

(giving rise to stalk disconnection). A pituitary MRI provides more information than a CT head scan.

5 She is likely to be growth hormone deficient and may benefit from treatment.

Answers to Question 22
F, F, T, F, F

A The presence of carcinoid syndrome implies that the gastrointestinal primary has metastasized to the liver.

B 5-HT is metabolized to 5-hydroxyindoleacetic acid, which can be measured in the urine.

C This is the basis for a radiolabelled octreotide scan and for treatment with somatostatin analogues.

D Octreotide therapy can give rise to gall stones.

E Survival is variable: patients with liver metastases may live for many years.

Answers to Question 23
F, F, T, F, T

A Elevated ACTH levels in Addison's disease lead to pigmentation (generalized, palmar creases, scars and buccal mucosa). Although vitiligo is a recognized association, it leads to areas of depigmentation.

B As a general rule, the final steroid dose of the day should be taken not later than 6.00 pm to mimic physiological glucocorticoid production and to avoid insomnia.

C Adrenal autoantibodies are positive in just over half of patients with Addison's disease of presumed autoimmune aetiology.

D In a suspected Addisonian crisis, the patient must be treated immediately with intravenous hydrocortisone after taking a single random cortisol sample. Definitive diagnostic tests should be deferred.

E Patients should be encouraged to do this: it is a very important safety precaution. However, in addition they must be advised to seek medical help for more serious illness or if there is diarrhoea or vomiting.

Answers to Question 24
1D 2F 3A 4E 5B 6C

1 A longer-acting preparation such as cabergoline can be used if a patient is unable to tolerate the side effects of bromocriptine.

2 Patients must be warned to report infections, especially a sore throat, and to attend their GP or hospital for an urgent neutrophil count.

3 All sulphonylureas can cause hypoglycaemia—glibenclamide is long acting and best avoided in the elderly.

4 Galactorrhoea, reflecting hyperprolactinaemia, may complicate treatment with antidopaminergic agents.

5 Amiodarone may cause hypo- or hyperthyroidism.

6 Desmopressin promotes water reabsorption in the distal renal tubule and collecting ducts and can lead to hyponatraemia if treatment is not carefully monitored.

Answers to Question 25

F, T, F, F, T

A Erectile dysfunction is a common disorder even outside the setting of diabetes mellitus, with the prevalence increasing with age.

B This suggests a psychogenic cause.

C Remember, sildenafil augments the erectile response to sexual stimulation.

D Only 5–10% of impotent patients are androgen deficient.

E Hyperprolactinaemia is a recognized cause of erectile dysfunction, and in the absence of a simple explanation (e.g. a mildly elevated level in a patient taking antidopaminergic treatment) should prompt a search to exclude associated pituitary disease.

Answers to Question 26

F, F, T, F, F

A Spermatogenesis requires specialist fertility treatment.

C If thyroid hormone replacement is given before adrenal insufficiency has been corrected, there is a significant risk of precipitating a hypoadrenal crisis.

D Men require testosterone to prevent the development of osteoporosis.

E Lower dose postmenopausal hormone replacement therapy preparations are more appropriate.

Answers to Question 27

A

The T1-weighted coronal MRI scan demonstrates a normal sized pituitary gland with a centrally located pituitary stalk. The appearances are not suggestive of a micro- or macro-adenoma and there is no evidence of haemorrhage. Although a normal scan does not exclude the possibility of a micro-prolactinoma, other causes of mild hyperprolactinaemia should be sought (preferably before undertaking the scan!).

Answers to Question 28

F, F, F, T, T

A Investigations should be initiated at 14 years of age in girls and $14\frac{1}{2}$ years in boys to exclude an underlying cause.

B Sex hormone treatment may accelerate pubertal development, and if the diagnosis is correct, then the child's own pubertal development will often take over.

C The normal consonance between sexual development and the growth spurt is preserved.

Answers to Question 29

A Haemochromatosis.

B Although a liver biopsy would confirm the diagnosis and allow the extent of iron deposition to be determined, some centres now offer genetic screening for the common Cys282Tyr mutation in the first instance. The finding of an elevated serum ferritin level is not diagnostic of haemochromatosis.

C Regular venesection until iron depletion is demonstrated by normalization of the serum ferritin level and transferrin saturation.

Answers to Question 30

T, F, F, T, F

A, B The retinal appearances are those of diabetic maculopathy (classical circinate macular exudates) and background retinopathy (microaneurysms, dot and blot haemorrhages). Maculopathy represents the commonest threat to vision in type 2 diabetics. Prompt referral to an ophthalmologist is necessary, in addition to correcting poor glycaemic control and hypertension.

C Although insulin therapy may be required to improve glycaemic control, it is commonly associated with weight gain rather than weight loss.

D The United Kingdom Prospective Diabetes Study (UKPDS) demonstrated the β-blocker atenolol to be as efficacious as the ACE inhibitor captopril in reducing micro- and macrovascular endpoints in type 2 diabetes. However, in this particular case, treatment with a β-blocker may exacerbate both his peripheral vascular disease and his erectile dysfunction.

E Contraindications to the use of sildenafil include nitrate therapy, significant cardiovascular disease and retinitis pigmentosa. The clinical finding of absent peripheral pulses is suggestive of significant peripheral vascular disease and is likely to be associated with coronary artery disease.

Answers to Question 31

F, T, F, F, F

A, D Treatment for hypothyroidism is essentially the same as in non-pregnant subjects, although thyroxine requirements usually increase as the pregnancy progresses (by as much as 50–100% by the end of the third trimester).

B Women with unrecognized and/or untreated hypothyroidism are relatively infertile. Those who do achieve pregnancy have a higher incidence of miscarriage, congenital malformations and stillbirth.

C Maternal TSH does not cross the placenta and therefore elevated levels do not predispose to fetal thyrotoxicosis. The aim of thyroxine replacement therapy is to restore euthyroidism, and thereby avoid the complications outlined in B.

E In the UK autoimmune thyroid disease and previous treatment for thyrotoxicosis account for nearly 90% of cases of hypothyroidism.

Answers to Question 32

A

1 Acromegaly (failure of elevated basal growth hormone level to suppress following a glucose challenge).

2 Adrenal insufficiency (subnormal short Synacthen test).

3 Diabetes mellitus (on both the 0′ and 120′ glucose values from the OGTT).

B

1 Hyperprolactinaemia.

2 Hypogonadotrophic hypogonadism.

Note: the abnormalities of thyroid function are likely to indicate over-replacement with thyroxine.

Answers to Question 33

B, C, E

A The ITT may help to distinguish true Cushing's syndrome from pseudo-Cushing's syndrome, but is not useful in discriminating between the causes of the former.

B The majority of corticotroph adenomas retain sensitivity to CRH unlike ectopic tumours.

C Selective venous sampling is an effective means of localizing the site of ACTH release.

D The low-dose dexamethasone test is used to screen for the presence of Cushing's syndrome but does not discriminate between the differing aetiologies. The high-dose dexamethasone test can help to distinguish between pituitary and ectopic ACTH secretion by virtue of the fact that the majority of pituitary tumours retain some sensitivity to glucocorticoid feedback.

E Ectopic ACTH secreting tumours predispose to hypokalaemia.

Answers to Question 34

A Free T_3 as the patient is likely to have T_3 toxicosis.

B Solitary toxic adenoma.

C Thyroid radioisotope scan.

D Although β-blockers may control the peripheral thyrotoxic effects, antithyroid drugs should be used to prepare the patient for definitive treatment with either surgery or radioactive iodine therapy.

Answers to Question 35

F, T, T, F, T

A Klinefelter's syndrome is a cause of male hypogonadism (the classical phenotype being associated with an XXY genotype).

B The majority of females with Turner's syndrome have gonadal dysgenesis with streak-like ovaries.

C Hyperprolactinaemia is associated with hypogonadotrophic hypogonadism by virtue of its ability to interfere with the normal function of the GnRH pulse generator.

D Hypothyroidism is classically associated with menorrhagia.

E Severe weight loss disrupts the normal function of the hypothalamo–pituitary–gonadal axis.

Answers to Question 36

A Excessive calorie intake.

B Supervised dietary modification with regular exercise.

Answers to Question 37

F

The appearances shown in Fig. 65 are typical of a com-

plete 3rd nerve palsy (note the complete ptosis, dilated pupil and abduction of the left eye whilst looking straight ahead). The coronal MRI scan of the pituitary fossa shows an area of haemorrhage within a pituitary macroadenoma. In the setting of the clinical presentation this is most likely to represent pituitary apoplexy complicated by the development of a complete 3rd nerve palsy.

Answers to Question 38

F, F, F, T, T

Both the 0 and 120 min glucose values are entirely normal. However, weight loss should still be recommended in light of the history of hypertension, and also to reduce the long-term risk of developing impaired glucose tolerance or frank diabetes.

Answers to Question 39

F, F, T, F, T

A These are non-specific findings reflecting enhanced sensitivity to circulating catecholamines.

B Surgery (e.g. hemi-thyroidectomy) or radioiodine are the preferred treatment options because of their potential to leave the patient euthyroid in the long term.

C The lack of uptake of radioisotope in thyroiditis contrasts with the enhanced uniform uptake typical of Graves' disease.

D Radioiodine is a safe and effective therapy for hyperthyroidism in patients under the age of 50 provided that there are no other contraindications to its use, e.g. pregnancy.

E Amiodarone is associated with both thyrotoxicosis and hypothyroidism.

Answers to Question 40

A Multiple myeloma.

B Full blood count—for anaemia; serum and urine electrophoresis—for paraproteinaemia; skeletal survey—for evidence of lytic bone lesions.

C Rehydration with intravenous normal saline followed by frusemide and intravenous pamidronate.

Notes: In multiple myeloma there is evidence of generalized osteoclast activation, marked by hypercalcaemia. As PTH levels are suppressed and there is no production of PTHrP, renal phosphate excretion is not increased, and accordingly serum phosphate levels are elevated. Treatment is as for severe hypercalcaemia of any cause, with treatment of the underlying myeloma.

Answers to Question 41

F, T, T, F, F

A Although osteoporosis is commoner in women, it is certainly not rare in men.

B Hyperthyroidism is one of the many secondary causes of osteoporosis and should always be excluded.

C Osteoporosis can cause back pain, even without evidence of fracture.

D Identifying patients at risk of osteoporotic fracture (primary prevention) is the major challenge in osteoporosis; treatment should be started in any patient with proven osteoporosis to reduce the morbidity associated with fracture.

E Osteoporosis can be caused by hyperparathyroidism; hypercalcaemia should therefore be excluded before calcium supplements are started. Alternative treatments may be more appropriate according to clinical circumstances.

Answers to Question 42

1C 2G 3F 4B

1 Tendon xanthomata are a marker of prolonged elevated levels of LDL cholesterol; to appear as early as 15 years of age, it is likely that the patient has homozygous familial hypercholesterolaemia in which LDL cholesterol may be as high as 20 mmol/L in adolescence.

2 Xanthelasmata typically appear in patients with long-standing elevations of LDL cholesterol; the additional presence of jaundice suggests cholestasis, e.g. primary biliary cirrhosis.

3 The genetic defect underlying Type III hyperlipoproteinaemia is inherited in an autosomal recessive manner; additionally, some environmental factor is required, so there is often no family history of dyslipidaemia or premature vascular disease.

4 Nephrotic syndrome produces a mixed hyperlipidaemia that is difficult to treat, as well as signs of hypoalbuminaemia due to the marked proteinuria.

Answers to Question 43

1B 2F 3GHJ 4K

Note: In addition, alcohol should be avoided, and no form of oral contraception is safe.

Answers to Question 44

A Type 1 diabetes, which can be confirmed by a fasting venous plasma glucose of 7.0 mmol/L or higher, or a random venous glucose of 11.1 mmol/L or higher.

B In type 1 diabetes there is complete lack of insulin as a result of destruction of the β cells of the islets of Langerhans in the pancreas. There is evidence implicating genetic factors, viruses and autoimmune processes in the development of this disorder.

C As there is complete insulin deficiency, treatment is required immediately. The patient should be educated in the administration of insulin and in home monitoring of blood glucose. Involvement of the entire diabetic team is helpful, as are the information booklets and diabetic camps organized by Diabetes UK.

Answers to Question 45

1A 2C 3E 4E

1, 2 A 3-month trial of a low-carbohydrate, low-fat diet is appropriate in almost all newly diagnosed type 2 diabetics. Where such dietary modification fails, treatment with a biguanide or a sulphonylurea should then be started, usually beginning with metformin in an obese patient.

3 Trials have shown that ACE inhibitors reduce the risk of progression to overt renal disease in diabetics with persistent microalbuminuria.

4 Hypertension should be rigorously treated in all diabetics; combination therapy will often be required but ACE inhibitors form an ideal first-line agent. β-Blockers are also effective but may exacerbate erectile dysfunction.

The Medical Masterclass series

4.4 Non-dose-related adverse drug reactions

4.5 Adverse reactions caused by long-term effects of drugs

4.6 Adverse reactions caused by delayed effects of drugs

4.7 Teratogenic effects

5 Prescribing in special circumstances

  5.1 Introduction

  5.2 Prescribing and liver disease

  5.3 Prescribing in pregnancy

  5.4 Prescribing for women of child-bearing potential

  5.5 Prescribing to lactating mothers

  5.6 Prescribing in renal disease

6 Drug development and rational prescribing

  6.1 Drug development

    6.1.1 Identifying molecules for development as drugs

    6.1.2 Clinical trials: from drug to medicine

  6.2 Rational prescribing

    6.2.1 Clinical governance and rational prescribing

    6.2.2 Rational prescribing, irrational patients?

Clinical Skills

General Clinical Issues

1 The importance of general clinical issues

2 History and examination

3 Communication skills

4 Being a doctor

  4.1 Team work and errors

  4.2 The 'modern' health service

  4.3 Rationing beds

  4.4 Stress

Pain Relief and Palliative Care

1 Clinical presentations

  1.1 Back pain

  1.2 Nausea and vomiting

  1.3 Breathlessness

  1.4 Confusion

2 Diseases and treatments

  2.1 Pain

  2.2 Breathlessness

  2.3 Nausea and vomiting

  2.4 Bowel obstruction

  2.5 Constipation

  2.6 Depression

  2.7 Anxiety

  2.8 Confusion

  2.9 The dying patient: terminal phase

  2.10 Palliative care services in the community

Medicine for the Elderly

1 Clinical presentations

  1.1 Frequent falls

  1.2 Sudden onset of confusion

  1.3 Urinary incontinence and immobility

  1.4 Collapse

  1.5 Vague aches and pains

  1.6 Swollen legs and back pain

  1.7 Gradual decline

2 Diseases and treatments

  2.1 Why elderly patients are different

  2.2 General approach to managment

  2.3 Falls

  2.4 Urinary and faecal incontinence

    2.4.1 Urinary incontinence

    2.4.2 Faecal incontinence

  2.5 Hypothermia

  2.6 Drugs in elderly people

  2.7 Dementia

  2.8 Rehabilitation

  2.9 Aids and appliances

  2.10 Hearing impairment

  2.11 Nutrition

  2.12 Benefits

  2.13 Legal aspects of elderly care

3 Investigations and practical procedures

  3.1 Diagnosis vs common sense

  3.2 Assessment of cognition, mood and function

Emergency Medicine

1 Clinical presentations

  1.1 Cardiac arrest

  1.2 Collapse with hypotension

  1.3 Central chest pain

  1.4 Tachyarrythmia

  1.5 Nocturnal dyspnoea

  1.6 Bradydysrhythmia

  1.7 Acute severe asthma

  1.8 Pleurisy

  1.9 Community-acquired pneumonia

  1.10 Chronic airways obstruction

  1.11 Upper gastrointestinal haemorrhage

  1.12 Bloody diarrhoea

  1.13 'The medical abdomen'

  1.14 Hepatic encephalopathy/alcohol withdrawal

  1.15 Renal failure, fluid overload and hyperkalaemia

  1.16 Diabetic ketoacidosis

  1.17 Hypoglycaemia

  1.18 Hypercalcaemia and hyponatraemia

  1.19 Metabolic acidosis

  1.20 An endocrine crisis

  1.21 Another endocrine crisis

  1.22 Severe headache with meningism

  1.23 Acute spastic paraparesis

  1.24 Status epilepticus

  1.25 Stroke

  1.26 Coma

  1.27 Fever in a returning traveller

  1.28 Septicaemia

  1.29 Anaphylaxis

2 Diseases and treatments

  2.1 Overdoses

Infectious Diseases and Dermatology

Infectious Diseases

Dermatology

1 Clinical presentations
  1.1 Blistering disorders
  1.2 Acute generalized rashes
  1.3 Erythroderma
  1.4 A chronic, red facial rash
  1.5 Pruritus
  1.6 Alopecia
  1.7 Abnormal skin pigmentation
  1.8 Patches and plaques on the lower legs
2 Diseases and treatments
  2.1 Alopecia areata
  2.2 Bullous pemphigoid and pemphigoid gestationis
  2.3 Dermatomyositis
  2.4 Mycosis fungoides and Sézary syndrome
  2.5 Dermatitis herpetiformis
  2.6 Drug eruptions
  2.7 Atopic eczema
  2.8 Contact dermatitis
  2.9 Erythema multiforme, Stevens–Johnson syndrome, toxic epidermal necrolysis
  2.10 Erythema nodosum
  2.11 Lichen planus
  2.12 Pemphigus vulgaris
  2.13 Superficial fungal infections
  2.14 Psoriasis
  2.15 Scabies
  2.16 Urticaria and angio-oedema
  2.17 Vitiligo
  2.18 Pyoderma gangrenosum
  2.19 Cutaneous vasculitis
  2.20 Acanthosis nigricans
3 Investigations and practical procedures
  3.1 Skin biopsy
  3.2 Direct and indirect immunofluorescence
  3.3 Patch testing
  3.4 Topical therapy: corticosteroids
  3.5 Phototherapy
  3.6 Systemic retinoids

Haematology and Oncology

Haematology

1 Clinical presentations
  1.1 Microcytic hypochromic anaemia
  1.2 Chest syndrome in sickle cell disease
  1.3 Normocytic anaemia
  1.4 Macrocytic anaemia
  1.5 Hereditary spherocytosis and failure to thrive
  1.6 Neutropenia
  1.7 Pancytopenia
  1.8 Thrombocytopenia and purpura
  1.9 Leucocytosis
  1.10 Lymphocytosis and anaemia
  1.11 Spontaneous bleeding and weight loss
  1.12 Menorrhagia and anaemia
  1.13 Thromboembolism and fetal loss
  1.14 Polycythaemia
  1.15 Bone pain and hypercalcaemia
  1.16 Cervical lymphadenopathy and weight loss
  1.17 Isolated splenomegaly
  1.18 Inflammatory bowel disease with thrombocytosis
  1.19 Transfusion reaction
  1.20 Recurrent deep venous thrombosis
2 Diseases and treatments
  2.1 Causes of anaemia
    2.1.1 Thalassaemia syndromes
    2.1.2 Sickle cell syndromes
    2.1.3 Enzyme defects
    2.1.4 Membrane defects
    2.1.5 Iron metabolism and iron-deficiency anaemia
    2.1.6 Vitamin B_{12} and folate metabolism and deficiency
    2.1.7 Acquired haemolytic anaemia
    2.1.8 Bone-marrow failure and infiltration
  2.2 Haemic malignancy
    2.2.1 Multiple myeloma
    2.2.2 Acute leukaemia—acute lymphoblastic leukaemia and acute myeloid leukaemia
    2.2.3 Chronic lymphocytic leukaemia
    2.2.4 Chronic myeloid leukaemia
    2.2.5 Malignant lymphomas—non-Hodgkin's lymphoma and Hodgkin's disease
    2.2.6 Myelodysplastic syndromes
    2.2.7 Non-leukaemic myeloproliferative disorders
    2.2.8 Amyloidosis
  2.3 Bleeding disorders
    2.3.1 Inherited bleeding disorders
    2.3.2 Acquired bleeding disorders
    2.3.3 Idiopathic thrombocytopenic purpura
  2.4 Thrombotic disorders
    2.4.1 Inherited thrombotic disease
    2.4.2 Acquired thrombotic disease
  2.5 Clinical use of blood products
  2.6 Haematological features of systemic disease
  2.7 Haematology of pregnancy
  2.8 Iron overload
  2.9 Chemotherapy and related therapies
  2.10 Principles of bone-marrow and peripheral blood stem-cell transplantation
3 Investigations and practical procedures
  3.1 The full blood count and film
  3.2 Bone-marrow examination
  3.3 Clotting screen
  3.4 Coombs' test (direct antiglobulin test)
  3.5 Erythrocyte sedimentation rate vs plasma viscosity
  3.6 Therapeutic anticoagulation

Oncology

1 Clinical presentations
  1.1 A lump in the neck
  1.2 Breathlessness and a pelvic mass
  1.3 Breast cancer and headache
    1.3.1 Metastatic disease
  1.4 Cough and weakness
    1.4.1 Paraneoplastic conditions

Cardiology and Respiratory Medicine

Cardiology

Neurology, Ophthalmology and Psychiatry

Neurology

Nephrology

Rheumatology and Clinical Immunology

Index

visual fields, hyperprolactinaemia
52
vitamin D
calcium regulation 97
deficiency 37, 91
hypercalcaemia 7, 97, 98
hypocalcaemia 99
metabolism *92*
osteomalacia 38, 91, 92, 93
supplements 8, 93, 38
volume status 5
vomiting 44
von Hippel–Lindau syndrome
65

water deprivation test 124
water intoxication, compulsive 9, 10
weakness
examination 37–8
hypokalaemia 40
neurological cause 37
proximal myopathy 36
weight loss 28–30, *31*
amenorrhoea 18
bulimia 44
causes 29
diabetes mellitus 101
HIV infection 30
investigations 30

management 30
nausea 44
polycystic ovarian syndrome 17, 79
reproductive disorders 79
tiredness and amenorrhoea 44–6
vomiting 44
see also Addison's disease; anorexia nervosa;
lymphoma
Wermer's syndrome **115**

xanthelasma *39, 86*
xanthomata *86*

Y chromosome, cryptic 21